THE
HAIRSTYLE
& HAIRCARE
BOOK

BY LINDA SONNTAG

CHARTWELL
BOOKS, INC.

A QUINTET BOOK

ISBN: 0-7858-0343-2

This book was designed and produced by
Quintet Publishing Limited
6, Blundell Street
London N7 9BH

Designers: Bobby Colgate–Stone and Neil Studwick
Mixed Media Picture Researcher: Vivian Adelman
Jacket Design: Nik Morley

Typeset in Great Britain by
Leaper and Gard, Bristol
Manufactured in China by
Regent Publishing Services Limited.

This edition produced for sale in the USA,
its territories and dependencies only.

Published by Chartwell Books
A Division of Book Sales, Inc.
P.O. Box 7100
Edison, New Jersey 08818–7100

Contents

Chapter 1
Hair Facts 4

Chapter 2
Your Hair 6

Chapter 3
Hair Care at Home 8

Chapter 4
Looking After Problem Hair 12

Chapter 5
Coloring Your Hair 16

Chapter 6
Hair Styles 24

Hair

Your hair is a valuable natural fibre and to get it looking at its best you should treat it with as much care as you would silk or wool. Fortunately, hair is very resilient. It is as strong as aluminium, and an average single hair can withstand a pull of 200g, which would snap most textile fibres. A healthy hair can be stretched by one fifth its normal length before breaking. If your hair is in poor condition because of neglect, or if it has been subjected to harsh treatment, all is not lost. With care and attention you will be able to restore its bounce and glossy sheen.

Hair grows all over the body except on the palms of the hands and the soles of the feet. The average adult scalp sprouts about 100,000 hairs; it is hair colour that determines the quantity. Redheads have thick hair, but the smallest number of strands. Next come brunettes. Blondes, who have the finest hair, have the greatest number of strands — up to 150,000. Black hair is the coarsest of all — the diameter of one black hair can be three times that of a blonde hair.

A single hair lives and grows for between two and six years — and in some cases, up to 20 — though, technically speaking, the hair shaft is dead matter, and only the root is alive. The shaft emerges from the papilla, a nodule at the base of the hair follicle below the surface of the skin. Hair growth cannot be stopped if a hair is pulled out by the root, because the papilla will eventually produce a new hair. The shape of the follicle determines the shape of the hair. A round follicle will produce straight hair that will usually grow long; an oval follicle produces wavy, medium-length hair, and a kidney-shaped follicle, most often found in black-skinned people, produces hair that is woolly and wiry and usually short.

Hair is 97 per cent protein and 3 per cent moisture, so the importance of protein in the diet for healthy hair is obvious. Each hair is made up of three layers. The inner core or medulla is the 'marrow' of the hair and is soft and spongy. It can deteriorate in old age and be damaged by drugs and chemicals. In some cases it is missing altogether and the hair becomes thin and brittle. The medulla is surrounded by the cortex, which is composed of long, thin, fibrous cells that give the hair its elasticity. The cortex contains the pigment that gives the hair its natural colour.

Pigments are red, yellow and black, and a mixture of these over the entire head gives the hair its individual shade. If no pigment is present, the hair is white. There is no such thing as grey hair — this is an illusion caused by white hairs appearing amongst hairs of the original colour. The cortex is the part of the hair that responds to chemicals intended to permanently curl, straighten or colour it.

The outer layer, the cuticle, is formed of hard scales of keratin, a protein, that overlaps like tiles on a roof. The cuticle protects the hair shaft. When the scales are lying smoothly, they reflect the light and give the hair its shine; they also trap the oil that gives the hair its lustre This oil, or sebum, the hair's natural conditioner, is produced by the sebaceous gland attached to the hair follicle. The hair is lubricated as more sebum is produced, but the ends of longer hair will never be reached — you will need to

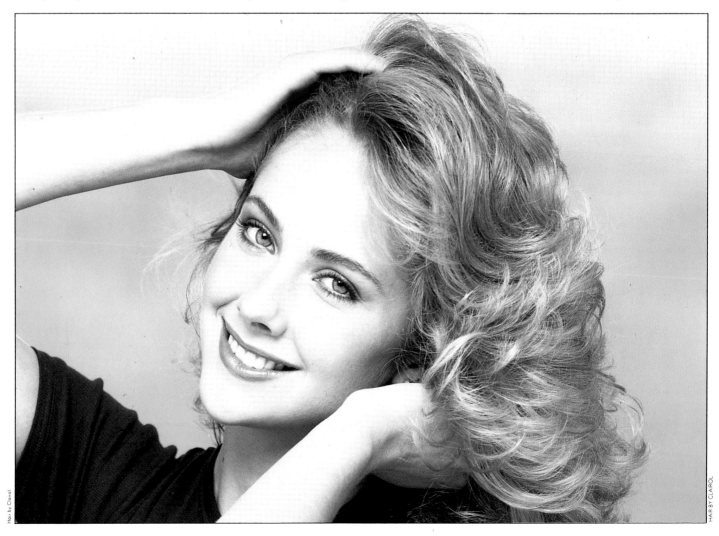

use a conditioner and trim off split ends. Lubrication is also stimulated by the tiny muscles around the follicle. It is these muscles that are responsible for the hair 'standing on end' through cold or fear.

Hair begins to grow before birth, but it is a myth that it continues to grow after death. It is the last part of the body to decay Everyone loses, on average, 50 hairs a day, and these are replaced, except in the case of thinning hair, by new growth. Hair grows at the rate of about 1cm per month. Strangely, it grows faster in summer than in winter, and faster during the day than at night. Women's hair grows faster than men's. Cutting hair does not accelerate growth, though shaving hair under the arms and on the legs may make it appear coarser because it then grows with a blunted end.

A baby may be born with very little hair, or with a lot. Its hair may fall out in the first weeks of life and then begin to grow again, and its hair type and colour may change. But by the time a child is about three, it will have settled down with the hair it will grow up with. A baby's head should always be washed along with the rest of its body at bath time. Avoid putting pressure on the soft crown of the head, but wash it gently to prevent the formation of a scaly condition called cradle cap. If this does appear, it can be treated with cotton wool soaked in warm oil to soften it before washing in the normal way.

Children's hair is as easily affected by diet as adults' hair is. Encourage your child to eat fresh fruit and vegetables, and to avoid sweet and greasy foods.

Hormonal changes in the body and an active lifestyle are often the cause of lank and greasy hair in teenagers. A diet that is low in fats, sugar and carbohydrates should be encouraged. Adolescents should also be encouraged to wash their hair as often as they want — even twice a day won't harm the hair, as long as a gentle shampoo is used and the hair is allowed to dry naturally. Conditioner need be applied only at the ends of long hair.

Dandruff is another problem that can arise during the teens. If frequent and thorough shampooing with a mild shampoo does not help, try a medicated brand. Dandruff in the teens is sometimes caused by dirt, grease and shampoo being left behind on the scalp. Wash and rinse the scalp carefully. If the problem persists, consult a trichologist.

Split ends should be trimmed off. These can be exacerbated by the excessive use of hairdriers and heated styling equipment.

During the 20s, when life gets into full swing, it may be tempting to take advantage of the fact that your hair is enjoying maximum health and expect it to bounce back of its own accord every time you perm or colour it, or every time you expose it to holiday sun or the chlorine of a swimming pool. Use a nourishing conditioner on damaged hair or rub in warm olive oil or a wax cream, then wrap your head in plastic film, tie it in a scarf and leave it for as long as you can — overnight if possible. Protect your hair from the sun under a hat or scarf. If you go swimming, always rinse salt water or chlorine out of your hair straight away, then shampoo and condition. A conditioning gel is an excellent idea for keen swimmers and sunbathers. Apply it generously to your hair before you go to the beach to achieve a wet look that will be quite in place and will protect your hair all day.

Pregnancy affects the hair in different ways — sometimes it makes it more lustrous, but other women are less fortunate and find themselves losing quantities of hair. Some mothers-to-be find that their perm loses its bounce. Nothing can be done about this, but a healthy diet will ensure that the hair regains its former condition as soon as possible after the birth.

A common problem in the 30s is a tendency to dry and brittle hair. This is sometimes the result of years of perming and colouring, but it is more likely due to stress or a bad diet. A certain amount of drying up is inevitable as the body's functions begin to slow down and the production of sebum is reduced. This is the time, too, when most people discover their first grey hairs. These are actually white hairs, which look grey when mingled in with hairs of your natural colour. Many women in their 40s decide to disguise their grey hairs with a specially formulated rinse. At this age you should use a rich shampoo and pay special attention to conditioning — a wax or oil treatment once a week will bring back the life into your hair. Henna treatments restore the shine to dull hair, but use one without a colorant on grey or white hair, or you may be dazzled by the result.

During the menopause, hormonal imbalance and the emotional stress that often goes along with it can cause significant hair loss, while facial hair may coarsen or grow darker. Many women find hormone replacement therapy (HRT) keeps their hair in good condition and stops it falling out. At the same time it benefits the skin, slowing down the deepening of wrinkles. It has other advantages, in that it helps the flesh to stay firmer longer and the spine to stay erect, and a continued dose of oestrogen cuts down the risk of a heart attack.

Whether to opt for HRT or not is a decision for each woman to make in consultation with her doctor. If you decide against it, you should be able to avoid distressing hair loss by keeping to a healthy diet, taking frequent exercise to stimulate the circulation, keeping the scalp scrupulously clean and using nourishing conditioners.

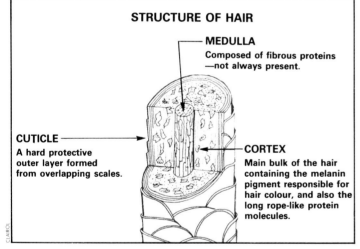

STRUCTURE OF HAIR

MEDULLA
Composed of fibrous proteins —not always present.

CUTICLE
A hard protective outer layer formed from overlapping scales.

CORTEX
Main bulk of the hair containing the melanin pigment responsible for hair colour, and also the long rope-like protein molecules.

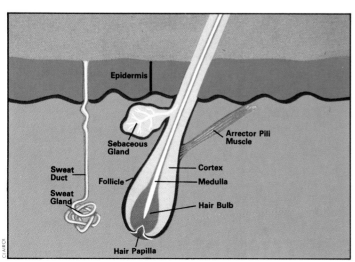

Epidermis

Sebaceous Gland

Arrector Pili Muscle

Sweat Duct

Follicle

Cortex

Medulla

Sweat Gland

Hair Bulb

Hair Papilla

Your Hair

A flattering hairstyle can be the most important single factor in your appearance. Not only does it tell about your character, it balances your body, frames your face and complements your clothes and lifestyle. A really professional haircut is a valuable investment, because it will make you feel good as well as look good.

When choosing a new hairstyle you should look carefully at the shape of your face. Try this when shampooing your hair. Lather it up onto the top of your head, put your glasses on if you wear them, and pull and pat it into different shapes.

• If you have an oval face, you are very lucky. Any style will suit you.
• A long face is best complemented by short hair that is quite full, with a fringe. Don't go for a severe long hairdo that will only accentuate the length of your face.
• If you have a round face, you should aim to add length. If you don't want long hair, part your hair on the side or add fullness on top. Avoid a neat bob with a fringe.
• All a square face needs is a little softening if the jawline is too heavy. Draw the attention away from the jaw with a diagonal fringe, soft tendrils of hair falling forward from the hairline and around the ears if you wear your hair up, or long loose hair with a bit of bounce below chin level.
• A heart-shaped face is also easy to flatter. All you need to do is avoid a heavy slab of a fringe that will make your face into a triangle. A softer fringe will help.
• Try a soft fringe too for a high forehead, or try a very heavy fridge that starts quite a way back and is 'V'-shaped, with the point of the 'V' in the centre of your forehead.
• If you have a receding or double chin, you need to draw attention away from it. Your hair will look best either piled to the top and back of your head, to balance the chin, or hanging loose to hide it.
• A large nose needs a short, fluffy style — anything sleek or straight will only over-emphasise it.

Once you have decided on the shape of style that will suit your face, you need to look at your hair type and see how the requirements of the one fit the potential of the other. Your hair may be thick or fine, curly or straight, and these factors will determine to a certain extent what you can do with it.

If you have thick or curly hair, you have plenty of natural volume to play with. Fine straight hair needs to be long, or permed, before you can achieve much volume — the sleek look is what comes naturally to you. However, the success of your hairstyle depends on the cut, and this can do much to offset any problems you may have with the nature of your hair.

Choosing a hairdresser

A really good hairdresser is not only an expert stylist — he or she will listen carefully to you, the client, will find out about your lifestyle — whether, for instance, you travel regularly to hot or humid climates or have the leisure to achieve a complicated hairstyle — and above all will look closely at your hair type and condition and advise you on both its potential and its limitations. A top hairdresser whose work you have admired in magazine photographs is not necessarily going to be the right one for you. It may not suit you to have the latest and most outrageous style that he or she has devised for a publicity shot — what you need is personal attention. A good hairdresser is one who will listen to your idea of how you want to look and study photographs of styles you like, and then explain how that style would look on you and also suggest modifications if necessary. A caring hairdresser will try to dissuade you from a drastic change of style or colour that would be wrong for your hair type, besides being expensive and bitterly regretted.

Take your time in settling down with a new hairdresser. A recommendation from a friend may encourage you to visit a new salon, where you can test the waters by having nothing more than a trim and blow-dry. Don't attempt to change your style on the first visit — wait until you're sure that you like the hairdresser's work. A visit to the salon should be a treat, not a chore. Choose somewhere with an atmosphere you like, where the staff are friendly and where the decor and music, if there is any, suit your mood. You want to be relaxed and you want to strike up a rapport with your hairdresser, even if conversation is minimal, otherwise you won't come out looking and feeling your best. It's important that you are punctual — you don't want your stylist to take revenge on your hair — and that if you're kept waiting you get an apology for the delay. Make sure, too, that you choose somewhere where brushes, towels and overalls are absolutely clean. There's nothing less appetising than someone else's dirty comb.

If you have enjoyed your first visit and you look and feel good, you may well have found a winner. Go back for a trim and perhaps a deep-conditioning treatment once a month until you feel confident that your hairdresser understands you and your hair. Only after this trial period should you change your style. Now you'll be looking forward to the results, not dreading them.

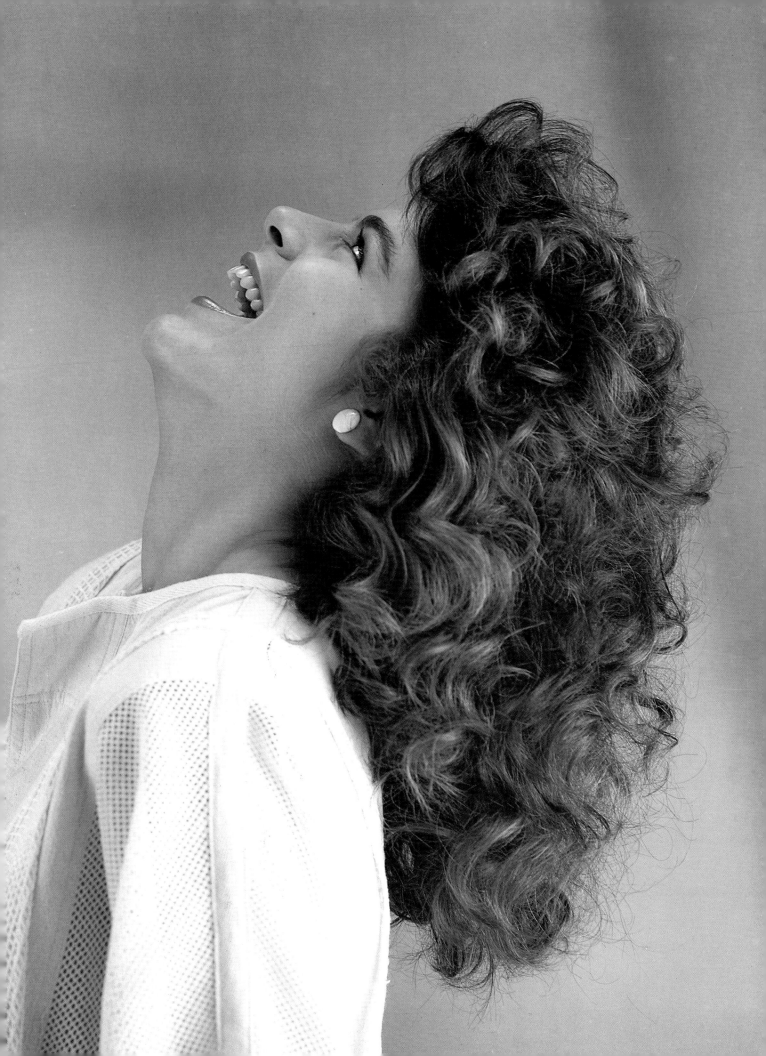

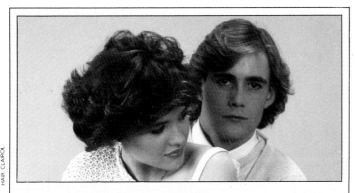

A career in hairdressing

Since Vidal Sassoon first appeared on the scene in the 1960s, hairdressing has not only been big business, it has become a field in which personalities achieve stardom and top salons become famous for their individual styling techniques. A successful stylist can make a career on board a luxury liner or travel the world working on photographic sessions for magazines. If you aim to own your own salon, and have an aptitude for stock control, budgeting, advertising and promotion as well as creative styling, there will be openings for you in management.

As in any career, experience is absolutely vital before you can succeed — and in hairdressing it takes a long time to get there. You have to be really dedicated to be willing to stand on the side-lines for so long, sweeping the floor, bringing clients their coffee, shampooing and handing perm papers and scissors to the stylist. But there is a short cut, and this is to go to a hairdressing school. A beginners' course usually lasts about six months and is expensive. Some fees cover a personal set of hairdressing equipment.

The advantages are that you learn faster about every aspect of hairdressing, and though you won't be offered a top job as soon as you have finished your course, you will end up with a diploma that will drastically reduce the time you spend on your apprenticeship. Another point to bear in mind is that hairdressing salons will usually take on only young school leavers, but enrolment in a hairdressing school is not restricted by age, so a six month beginners' course could be your answer if you're looking for a change of career.

In most schools classes are kept small and tuition is intensive. Practical studies take place in salon conditions where cutting, perming, conditioning, colouring and blow-drying are demonstrated on live models. The theory of hair care and hair design, hygiene and salon etiquette are also included in the course — and some schools also run classes on make-up and manicure that can be very useful if you want to diversify.

Hairdressing is a career that you can succeed in wherever you live. It's hard work, but it's creative and it's a job in which you'll be likely to meet a great variety of people. Financial rewards can be high at the top, but wherever you work your greatest reward will be a satisfied client — someone who looks and feels good, thanks to your understanding and skill.

Hair Care at Home

Shampooing

However beautiful your hair is naturally, you need to treat it well, and the first essential is regular shampooing. How often you wash your hair depends entirely on you — wash it as often as you need to keep the scalp scrupulously clean. A mild pH-balanced shampoo correctly formulated for your hair type is best as it won't irritate the scalp or disturb the acid/alkaline balance of the hair. Don't be tempted to use detergents such as washing-up liquid as these will strip the hair of its natural oils. One shampoo will normally suffice. Using warm water from a spray, wet your hair thoroughly. Then pour a little shampoo into your cupped hand and massage it firmly but gently all over your scalp and through your hair. Rinse very thoroughly again from the spray, until the water runs from your hair perfectly free of soap.

In an emergency, you can use a dry shampoo — rub it into the hair and scalp, leave for a minute or two and then brush out — or dab your scalp and hair with cotton wool soaked in eau-de-cologne. Both methods get rid of grease, but of course neither is as satisfactory as a good wash. If you have run out of shampoo, try using the yolks of three eggs, beaten, instead.

Conditioning

There are three basic types of conditioner. A gentle cream moisturises and adds gloss. A rinse gets rid of static and makes hair more manageable. A deep-treatment conditioner nourishes and brings life back to dull or damaged hair. Deep wax or oil treatments should be left on the hair, under plastic film and a towel,

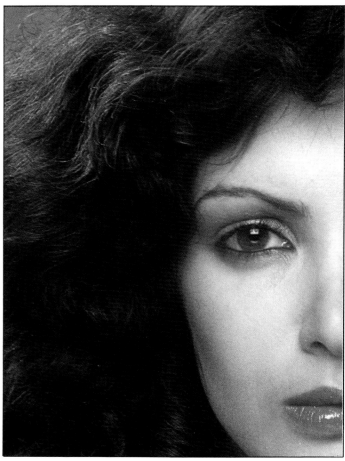

Healthy hair in top condition is your first beauty asset

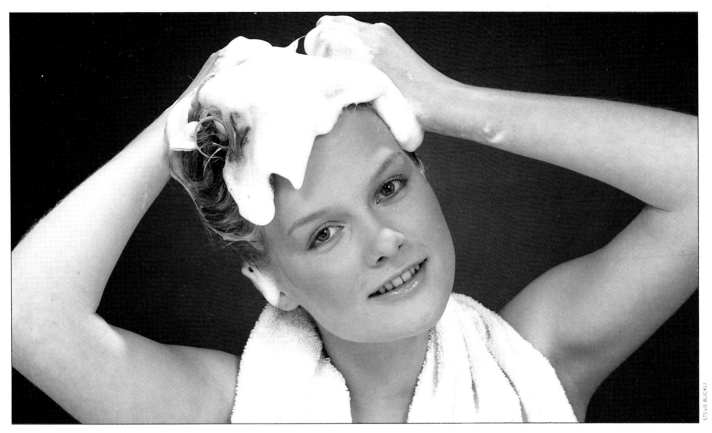

for as long as possible (overnight is ideal), and used once a week, or once a month, as necessary.

Ordinary conditioners, the creams and rinses, are applied in the same way as shampoo. Massage gently into the scalp and run your fingers through your hair so that it gets to the ends as well as the roots. Leave the conditioner on for a minute or two — perhaps while you soak in the bath or shower — then rinse thoroughly with warm water. A final cool-water rinse flattens the keratin scales on the hair shaft and makes the hair shinier.

You can make a herbal rinse for dark hair by immersing as much rosemary as you can find in water, bringing to the boil and leaving to steep overnight. Strain off the liquid and mix it half and half with cider vinegar. Use diluted with two parts of warm water. For fair or blonde hair, use camomile instead of rosemary.

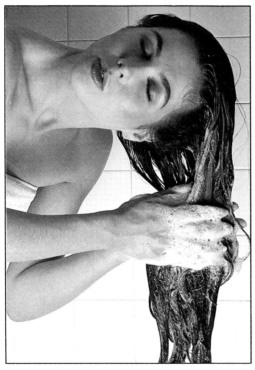

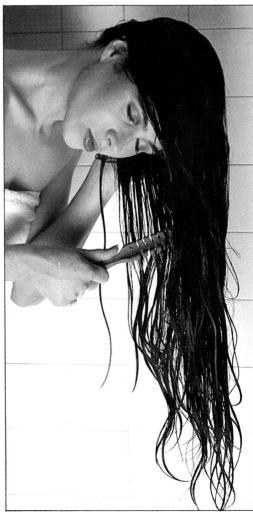

When you shampoo your hair, be thorough, but gentle. Work the lather in carefully, massaging the scalp with the fingertips. Rinse your hair with lukewarm water from a bathroom hose before conditioning. The tips of your hair, especially if it is long, will need particular attention. Rinse again, and wrap your hair in a towel

Drying

Whatever method you choose for drying your hair, you should first comb it through. Start at the tip, easing the tangles gently out, and work back along the hairshaft. If you start at the scalp, you'll only create fiercer tangles lower down. Take your time and don't tug — carelessness will damage your hair. Use a wide-toothed comb on wet hair — it will free the tangles more easily than a fine-toothed one. Leave your brush (if you use one at all — they often cause static) until your hair is dry. It will snarl wet hair and stretch it to breaking point.

The best way to dry your hair is to leave it and let it dry naturally. To add body and increase the manageability of fine hair, use a mousse or gel. Squirt the mousse or squeeze the gel onto a cupped hand. Rub your palms together, then spread the mousse or gel over the hair. Comb through into the style you want, or comb back from the face to give extra lift. Another way of giv-

Any hairstyle will hold better and last longer if you use a styling aid such as a mousse or gel

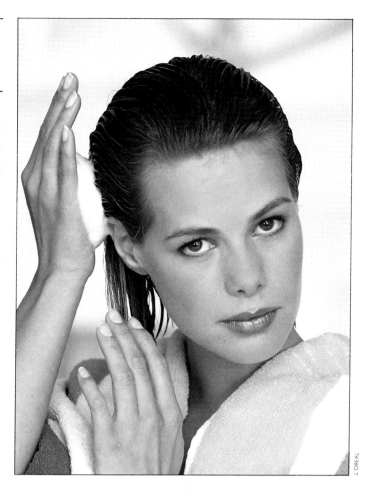

ing your hair a lift is to scrunch it up with your fingers as it dries. If you haven't the time to let your hair dry naturally, blot and squeeze dry with a towel before combing out. You can then set or blow dry.

To set, first apply the setting lotion of your choice, then divide your hair with a tail comb into even sections. Don't put too much hair on any one roller. Curly hair will get even curlier on small rollers — use larger ones for a healthy bounce. Thin hair needs to be rolled into a tighter curl on smaller rollers. Hold the hair away from the head at an angle of 90 degrees, and wind firmly, but without stretching, onto the roller. Secure with a pin. Use sellotape or clips for curls around the face. If you don't like the idea of rollers and pins, try the new 'shap-

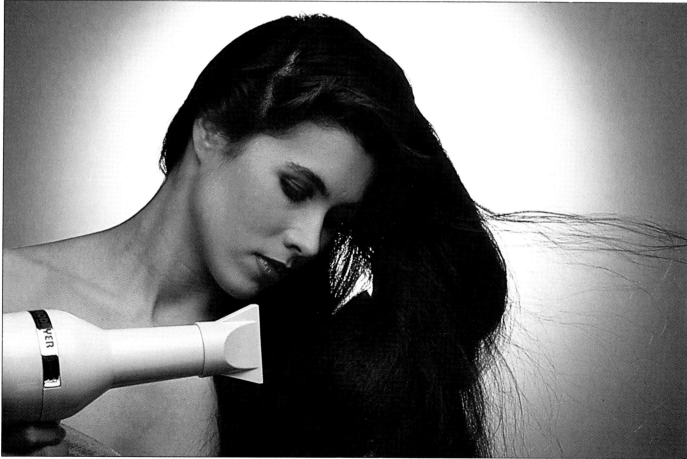

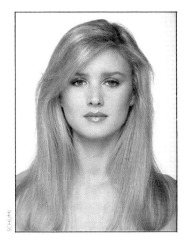

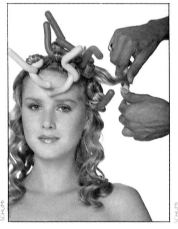

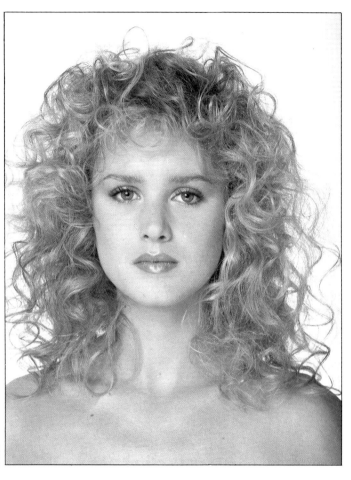

The model's long fine hair would be damaged by heated rollers and a perm would almost certainly cause it to break. When she wants a curly look the ideal way to achieve it is to use bendy shapers — the modern equivalent of rags. The hair is wrapped round the shapers while still slightly damp, then allowed to dry naturally. Shapers are simple to use. They are made of bendy lightweight foam and to secure them you just twist them over. They come in bright colours and look more decorative than rollers. They are heat resistant, so you can use a blow drier if you wish. When the hair is dry, unwind the shapers and fluff it out with the fingers.

Other ways of creating a curl are with more traditional rollers or with heated styling tongs. When using rollers, be careful not to put too much strain on the hair at the roots. If possible, allow the hair to dry naturally

ers'. They are bendy sticks round which you wind your hair. You then twist the shaper round on itself to hold the hair in place. Shapers act on the same principle as rags did, when they were used to curl Goldilocks-type hair. They are colourful and look pretty, which is more than can be said for rollers, so you won't feel embarrassed if you're interrupted wearing them.

If you set your hair, you should wait until it is completely dry before taking out the rollers. If you are sitting under a dryer, turn it off before your hair is quite dry and let the drying process finish naturally. Excessive heat is always damaging to the hair.

Comb each lock of hair through as you remove the rollers, starting at the nape of the neck and working up to the forehead. If the result is too hard and you can see the partings left by the rollers, you may need a little gentle back-brushing to disguise your handiwork, but be careful not to back-comb or brush too

vigorously, as this will break the hairshaft. A light hairspray applied directly from the aerosol, or sprayed onto a brush and run through the hair if your style is smooth and sleek, will help hold the shape longer.

Most modern styles rely not on a set, but on a superb cut and clever blow-drying. When a hairdresser blow-dries your hair it takes next to no time and looks very simple indeed, but as you will find when you start to do it yourself, it needs a little practice. Choose a plastic wand brush with widely spaced, springy bristles and hold it in your right hand if you are right-handed. Work from the nape, pinning the damp top hair on top of your head out of the way. Divide the hair into sections and wind it over the brush. Blow with the hairdrier from the root to the end of the strands. Don't hold it too close to the hair and keep it moving all the time, always in the direction of the hair growth. Work your way round the sides of your head and finish off with the crown.

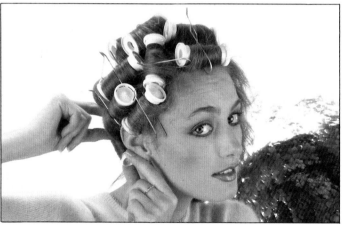

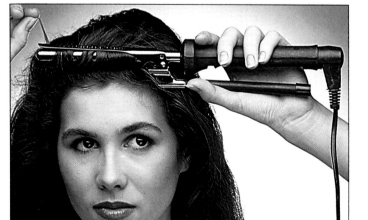

11

Looking After Problem Hair

Oily hair

The result of overactive sebaceous glands is oily hair and skin. Oily hair is most often fine hair, and this aggravates the problem of lank and lifeless locks. You should watch your diet and cut out greasy foods. Plenty of fresh fruit and salads with lots of mineral water to drink will help. It will come as a great relief to you to know that it is a fallacy that frequent shampooing makes the hair even more greasy. If you spent your adolescent years in misery because you were told you should only wash your hair every three days even though it was dreadfully greasy for two of them, then forget it. Your hair looks good only when it is clean, so wash it as often as you like — even twice a day if the weather is hot and sticky or very windy.

Use a mild shampoo and use a cream conditioner only at the ends of long hair. The best after-shampoo rinse for an oily head is an astringent one. Try a home-made herbal rinse or simply dilute some cider vinegar (stronger vinegars will have you smelling like a fish and chip shop) in luke-warm water and sluice it over your head after washing your hair. The acid in it will flatten the keratin scales on the hair-shaft and give extra shine as well as counteracting the grease.

Another very useful preparation for oily hair, especially when it is fine and flyaway too, is a hair gel or mousse. Even if you let your hair dry naturally after applying it, you will find it gives extra bounce and texture.

Dry hair

Dry hair is caused by under-active sebaceous glands or by over-exposure to wind, salt or chlorinated water or heat. Heat is the most common source of damage to the hair, whether from the sun, over-use of the hairdryer or heated styling appliances, or from central heating. Too frequent perming and bleaching also makes the hair brittle and unmanageable. If your hair has a constant tendency to break, apparently for none of these reasons, check with your doctor, as it may be due to drugs you are being prescribed.

Washing dry hair will not strip it of its natural oils, as it used to be thought. Whatever your hair type, your prime objective must be to keep it clean and if you use the correct products gently massaged into the scalp you will be able to restore shine to the driest hair. Use a rich shampoo, rinse clean with luke-warm water and follow with a cream conditioner, combing it through to the ends of the hair. Once a week, give yourself a warm olive oil or wax treatment. Massage it well into the scalp, comb the hair through and cover in cling film, then wrap in a towel or scarf. Leave it on for at least an hour, or overnight if you can. Wash out the oil with two latherings of shampoo and condition as normal. This treatment is especially good for bleached or heat-damaged hair.

Dandruff

The best treatment for dandruff is frequent shampooing with a mild shampoo. For a severe case of dandruff use a medicated shampoo. The most important thing is to keep the scalp scrupulously clean. Make sure that your diet is a healthy one and includes white meat or fish, eggs, cheese, fresh fruit and raw vegetables. Drink plenty of mineral water. Take exercise to help overcome tension. If dandruff persists, visit your doctor.

Excessive hair loss

Normally about 50 hairs will be lost from the head each

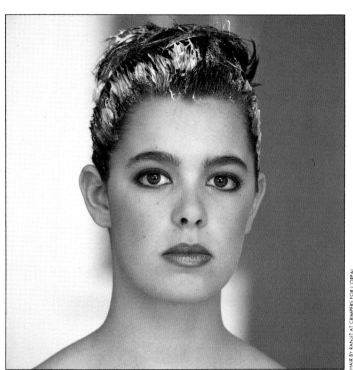

A regular deep-conditioning treatment is necessary to nourish dry hair and keep it glossy.

Condition your hair after every shampoo and deep-condition once a month

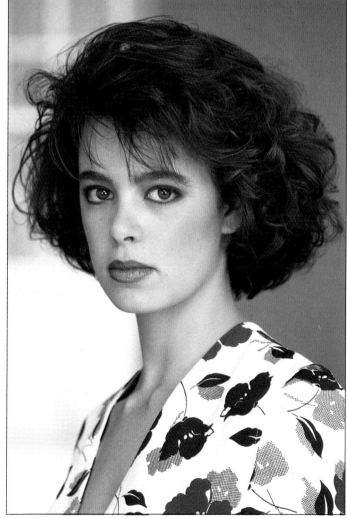

Long hair should be treated with the utmost care — avoid chemicals and heated appliances if you can. Pay special attention to the tips, which can be as much as six years old. Condition them and get them trimmed regularly to avoid unsightly split ends

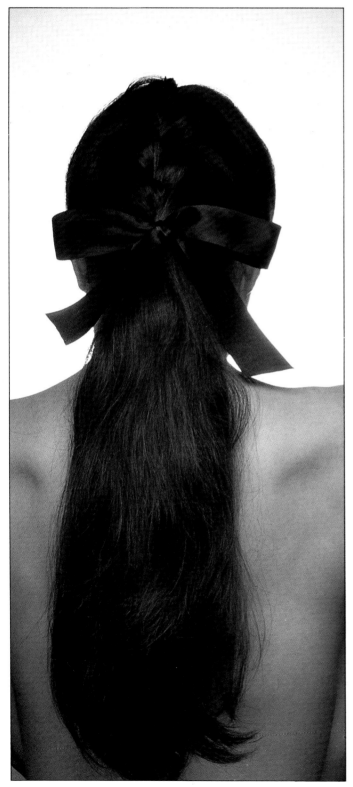

day. If your hair loss is more severe, the first thing to do is check your diet. Your hair will never be luxuriant if your diet is poor. Try to get plenty of fresh air and exercise, as well as lots of sleep. Use a comb, not a brush. Slightly more hair loss in spring and autumn is quite natural. Keep your hair short — it will look fuller and the weight of long hair may cause more of it to fall out. See your doctor or trichologist if you are upset by this problem.

Split and broken hair

If your hair is in very bad condition, splitting and breaking, it can be due to over-perming and bleaching, or to careless use of heated styling appliances or severe exposure to a merciless sun. Breaks and splits can never be mended, so your hair will need a good professional cut and regular trimming until new growth has replaced the damaged hair. In the meantime, treat your hair gently and give it a weekly deep-conditioning treatment to restore its shine. If you wish to perm or colour your hair yourself at this stage, take care to follow the manufacturer's instructions. If, when your hair is in better condition, you decide to perm or colour it professionally, always get your hairdresser to do a strand test first.

Keeping it long

Long hair is a valuable asset and needs to be treated very gently. If you are contemplating a change of colour, or a perm, always take your hairdresser's advice and don't attempt anything drastic at home.

To keep long hair in top condition and avoid broken and split ends, you will need to be aware that your number one enemy is heat. The tips of your hair are probably about four years old, and four years of regular treatment with hairdryers and various electrical styling appliances may often result in some damage. The ends of long hair should be trimmed regularly to remove split ends, and your hair should be allowed to dry naturally if possible. If you want to add bounce or curl without endangering your hair by constant use of heated rollers, try using bending shapers, or, if you can't find these in the shops, use the old-fashioned rag technique. Both work on the same principle — used on slightly damp hair they will give plenty of movement, while on dry hair they will give bounce. They are particularly effective when used in conjunction with a styling mousse. When you dress out the hair, finger the curls apart, starting from the nape and sides of the head and finishing with the crown. Brush through for a fluffier style.

More time-consuming, but very spectacular, is the pre-Raphaelite look. This is achieved by making tiny plaits — as many as you can manage — all over the head. It is best done on damp hair and left overnight. In the morning, undo the plaits and carefully finger through. Be sparing with your brush and comb if you want to keep the gently rippling curls in longer.

If you are prepared to spend some time perfecting your techniques with plaits, knots, buns and chignons, you can create a whole wardrobe of styles that will change your appearance as dramatically as a new outfit, but cost you next to nothing. Start with a simple pony tail, making sure that you always use a covered elastic band and remove it gently, and coil the hair this way and that to see what suits you. Enlist the aid of a few stylish combs and slides, and buy yourself a collection of pretty ribbons.

You may decide to adopt a new and sophisticated style for a special occasion. Experiment with it first! Don't leave it to the last minute: you may find it doesn't suit you at all, or that you feel self-conscious and unused to your new image — or even that your friends don't recognise you!

If the special occasion is your own wedding, then it's vital that you have a trial run. Your hairdresser will want to know the style of your dress, and headdress, if you are wearing one. Take your headdress along with you so that your hairdresser can show you how to secure it — the last thing you want on your wedding day is a hairstyle collapsing under the weight of yards of lace, or a veil that takes off at the slightest gust of wind.

Black Afro hair

The range of beauty products for black hair and the number of hairdressers who specialise in Afro styling has increased dramatically over the past 10 years. As with any other hair type, a balanced diet is needed for healthy hair, but black hair has extra requirements because it is coarse, fragile and dry and highly susceptible to atmospheric conditions.

Not so long ago, the answer to brittle, dull and unmanageable black hair used to be a thick coating of oil applied after infrequent washing. It was supposed to act as a straightener and a gloss. It had to be removed with a strong detergent shampoo as it clogged the hair follicles. The shampoo stripped the hair, undoing any good the oil might have done it, and irritated the scalp into the bargain. Hair loss and dandruff were often the results. Today's preparations are lighter and kinder to the hair and leave it looking clean and healthy.

Black hair should be washed as often as necessary with a mild shampoo. Always follow the shampoo with a conditioner, and give your hair a wax or oil deep-conditioning treatment every month or fortnight. For dry or irritated scalps there are special scalp conditioners. Moisturise your hair every day you don't wash it with one of the aerosol preparations available at your chemist. Because black hair is so sensitive to atmosphere and will lose moisture rapidly when it is dry and hot, and absorb moisture in damp conditions, so losing its style, you may find a reversion-resistant hair spray is a help. This will both hold your style and prevent excess loss of precious moisture — but use it sparingly to avoid a rigid look.

Get your hair trimmed regularly — black hair is wayward and needs constant taming as well as pampering. Many black women who don't like the limitations of the frizzy halo now sculpt their hair in a spectacular design of head-plaits.

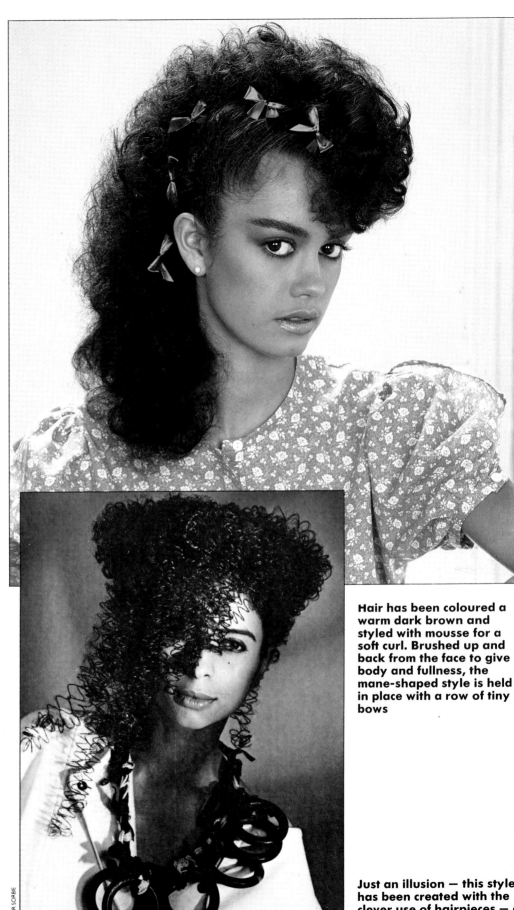

HAIR BY TREVOR SORBIE

Hair has been coloured a warm dark brown and styled with mousse for a soft curl. Brushed up and back from the face to give body and fullness, the mane-shaped style is held in place with a row of tiny bows

Just an illusion — this style has been created with the clever use of hairpieces — a stunning way of changing your looks without growing your hair long

This naturally curly hair is tinted arctic blonde above the temples and low-lighted for curl definition. The airy top is complimented by cropped sides and back for a triangular silhouette, defying the round head shape that holds most wearers of curly hair

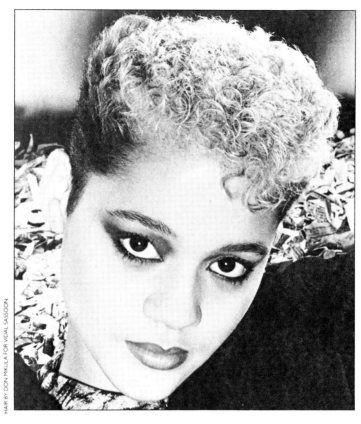

HAIR BY DON MIKULA FOR VIDAL SASSOON

Naturally curly hair has been straightened and tong-set for a fuller more bouyant curl. The auburn highlights follow the gentle upward movement of the front hair, while the back and sides are cropped short to create a neat head shape

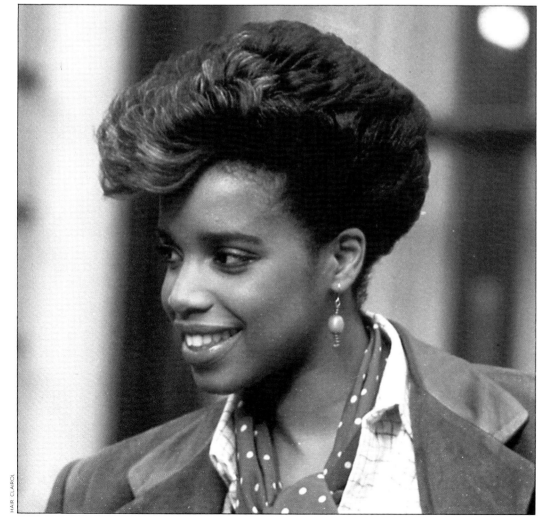

HAIR CLAIROL

This can be the most individual expression of your personality — it can be the height of elegance, intricately coiled and corn-rowed, or it can be a simple fringe of tiny plaits framing your face.

Another way to tame black hair is to straighten it. If you are wary of the damaging potential of chemical straightening on fragile hair, you can use a hot comb or curling tongs. The hair will need to be well conditioned before heat is applied. After washing, divide your hair into five sections — top, two sides, crown and nape. Twist and pin up each section out of the way. Beginning at the nape, apply concentrated scalp and hair conditioner. Comb a layer of the hair downwards, rub conditioner into the scalp with the fingertips, and comb it right through the hair, paying special attention to the ends. Gradually move round the sides and front of the head, finishing with the crown. It is a process that will take time, but the end result — glossy, well protected hair — will be well worth the effort.

Once the whole head has been conditioned, you can begin to go over the hair again, smoothing it out with the curling tongs or hot comb. Always use an appliance that is thermostatically controlled. When you have worked through each section and all the hair is straight, curl the hair into style on large rollers, or with the curling tongs.

For information on chemical straightening and a new soft curly perm for black hair, see the section on perming and straightening. If you want to colour your hair, you should seek the advice of a professional hairdresser. It is difficult to colour very curly hair yourself and harsh chemicals are not kind to dry, brittle hair or sensitive scalps. A semi-permanent rinse in a rich chestnut or deep brown can add depth and glow to your hair colour, and spray-on highlights and glitter look stunning for a temporary change of mood.

Colouring Your Hair

There are three different types of hair colour: temporary, semi-permanent and permanent.

Temporary colour

The mildest colourant you can use is the water rinse. This adds colour to the outer layer of the hair, the cuticle, which is then washed away with the next shampoo. It will also come off, of course, if you go out in the rain. Water rinses are useful to tone streaks of grey hair or to soften a too-brassy blond. Usually, no skin test is needed for water rinses. They are simple to use at home and usually applied after shampooing. The same effects can be achieved with coloured setting lotions, all-in-one shampoo/rinses, coloured sprays, gels or mousses.

Semi-permanent colour

Semi-permanents contain no bleaching agents and so cannot lighten the hair — they merely change its tone The colour does penetrate the cuticle temporarily, but is washed out after about half a dozen shampoos. A semi-permanent tint is useful for disguising grey hairs, giving depth to mousy hair and life to a dull blonde, or enriching brown hair with reddish tones. If you tint your hair at home, you will need to carry out a skin test 24 hours before you use the product on your hair. If you follow the manufacturer's instructions closely, you will give your hair added lustre as well as colour, because most contain an effective conditioner.

Permanent colour

Using a permanent tint is the only way to change your hair colour drastically. Exercise restraint if you want the results to look natural, and choose a tint that's only two or three shades lighter than your own colour. A strand test will help you decide if you've made the right choice. Don't chop a great chunk out of your hair for this — take about 50 hairs (which is after all only one day's natural hair loss) from all over your head. Follow the manufacturer's instructions and study the results in the sunlight. If you like what you see, hold the strand to your face and check that it doesn't clash with your complexion. Permanent tints are mixed with hydrogen peroxide and you should always carry out a skin test 24 hours in advance of using the product on your hair. If you are colouring your own hair, a good place to test the tint is on the tender skin inside the forearm. A hairdresser will normally do the test behind your ear, where it won't show if your skin reacts badly, but you need to do it somewhere where you can see it. Make sure not to wash the patch of skin you have tested, and if the product irritates your skin at all, don't use it.

Permanent tinting is a chemical process that works by lifting the overlapping keratin cells on the cuticle and penetrating the hairshaft. The bleach strips the hair of its natural colour and makes the cortex porous. The cortex then absorbs the new colour. Timing is crucial, and a professional colorist will be best able

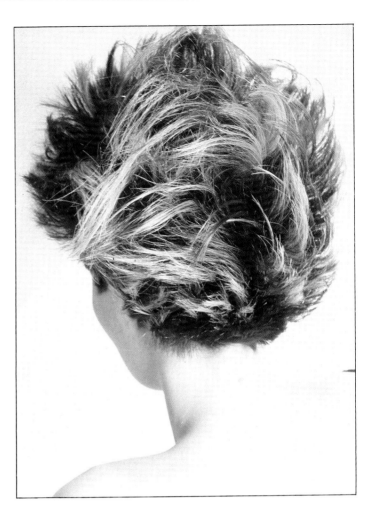

Imaginative colouring and styling have created this stunning effect. Two colours — red and white — have been applied to the hair. This has been repeated throughout the hair. The finished effect complements the cut and results in a superb dappled look

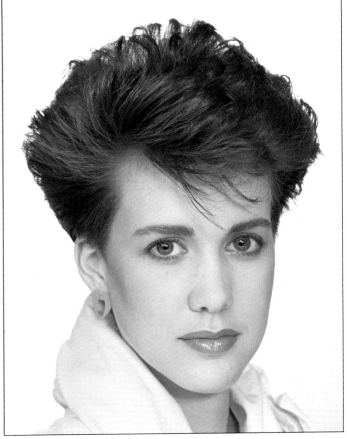

A hair colouring technique has been used to achieve a subtle blend of colour throughout the crown and forehead area. There is no methodical approach with this technique. Colour only as much hair as you feel emphasises the hair style. With this style the nape and the sides were left untreated to achieve a three-dimensional effect

HAIR BY RICHARD BRYANT OF SHAGGERS FOR L'OREAL

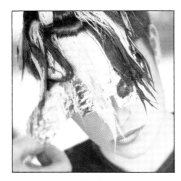

Using tin foil, three colours are applied to sections of the hair

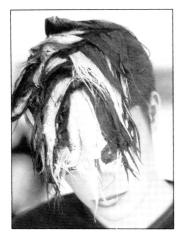

Each time a different colour order is used — white, red and black, the red, white and black, then black, white and red

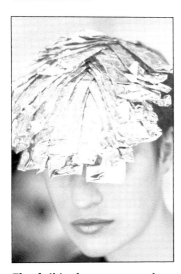

The foil is then wrapped firmly around the model's hair. The finished effect (right) is a unique marbling effect

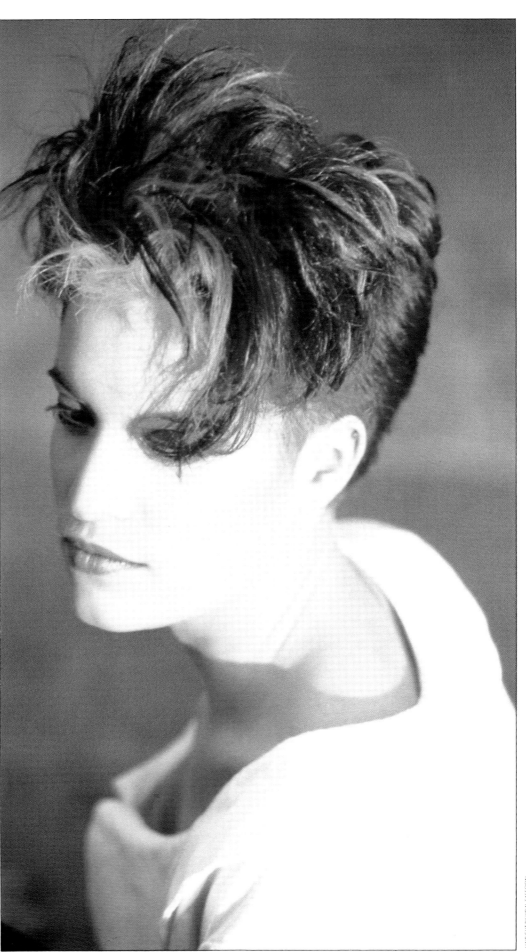

to judge how long to leave the colour on your particular hair type — finer hair takes less time to absorb the colour than coarser hair. Permanent tinting can go badly wrong, resulting in a surprising colour and damaged hair, if it is not done properly. If you choose to do it at home, make sure you follow the manufacturer's instructions exactly. Misuse of bleaching or permanent colouring may cause your hair to split and break. Your hairdresser may advise you to try a gentler method until your permanent colour has grown out.

Highlighting, streaking and tipping are sophisticated and selective forms of permanent colouring that require expert timing and blending. Nowadays they can be carried out at home. Professional highlighting is popular, though expensive, because it emphasises the nuances of colour in your hair, underlining its natural beauty. Strands of hair are drawn through holes in a plastic cap and treated with bleach or woven out and then wrapped in tin foil. The bleach is rinsed off when the desired colour has been reached, then the whole head is shampooed and conditioned, perhaps after having been treated with a semipermanent toner to blend the shades more subtly. Highlights grow out fairly naturally and need to be renewed only every three or four months.

In another process, bleach is painted in narrow stripes down the length of the hair. If you attempt this at home, you may end up looking like a zebra.

Tipping is exactly what it says — colouring just the ends of the hair. Often two or three shades of colour are used in all of these processes.

Vegetable dyes
Unlike chemical dyes these do not alter the structure of your hair. They are non-toxic, so no skin test is necessary. Vegetable dyes cling to the cuticle of the hair and leave it soft, shining and full of body —

so they are particularly useful on fine limp hair.

The most popular vegetable dye is henna, which has been used for thousands of years to give the hair rich red tones. There are different shades of henna available today — some of them compounded with other substances — and these are not compatible with any form of permanent hair colour or permanent wave. Always do a strand test, though the instruction leaflets that come with most brands of true red henna usually err on the cautious side where timing is concerned — in eastern countries women leave henna on their heads for 48 hours, basting occasionally with oil to stop it drying out.

Henna is the dried crushed leaves of the plant *Lawsonia alba*. It is mixed with hot water and a dash of lemon juice or vinegar and, for the most even results, painted onto the hair section by section. If you do this at home you will be bound to make a mess. Wear old clothes and be prepared to spend some time cleaning your bathroom afterwards. Pile the hennaed hair on top of your head, cleaning any henna off your skin with damp cotton wool (pay attention to the ears, too). Wrap a strip of cotton wool around the hairline to stop the dye running down your face and cover the head in cling film. Tie an old scarf or towel round your head. To speed up the colouring process, warm your head by using a hairdrier or sitting in the sun. When you decide your time is up, wash out the henna with several shampoos and rinse thoroughly with a bathroom spray. Your hair will be left in top condition, full and lustrous. Don't use henna on blonde, grey, white or chemically tinted hair, as the results will be unpredictable.

Other natural dyes can be made from infusions of camomile or marigold, both of which produce a subtle lightening effect, or from sage or walnut, which will give a soft brown tone to grey hair. Walnuts, if you use them, should be boiled for several hours.

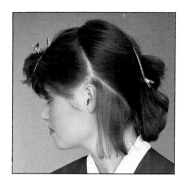

Divide the hair into two large sections from ear to ear and secure with clips

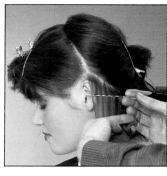

Take your first section diagonally on the hairline behind the ear

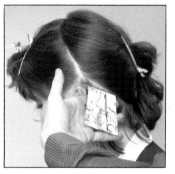

Alternate the colouring method: 1 Weave out and colour middle lengths; 2 Weave out and colour from

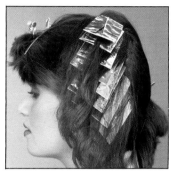

roots to tips; 3 Colour from roots to tips; 4 Colour entire section from roots to tips, working up to crown

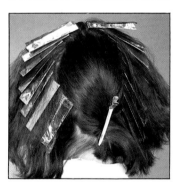

Complete the other side in the same way. Work up to join the crown on the back section

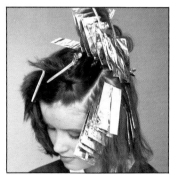

Divide the front into five sections back from hairline. Alternate the weave pattern as above

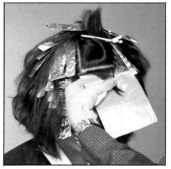

Take the next section above it and work backwards following the same method

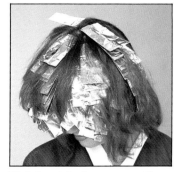

Finish with the top section, following the same method alternating the weave to give the result opposite

Reflective Lights

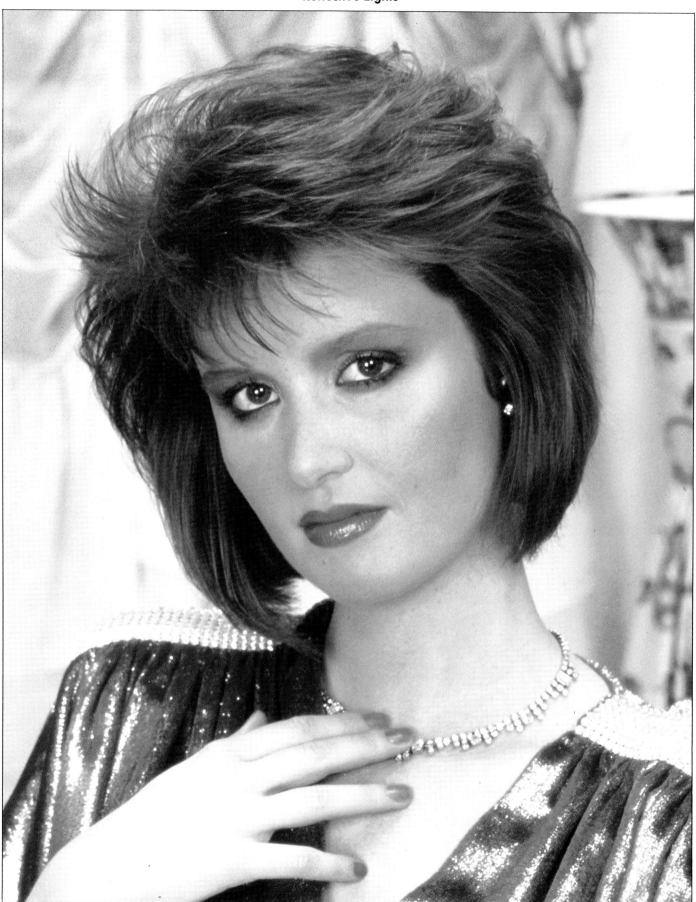

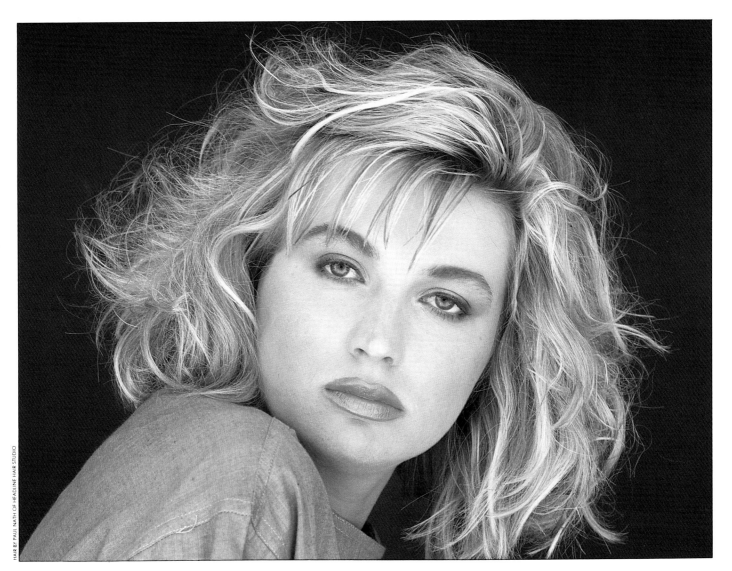

The two girls on these pages have had their hair tinted and highlighted by the method shown above right. Both styles show the advantage of highlighting to emphasise the movement of the hair, whether it is a soft easy curl or a more scrunched look

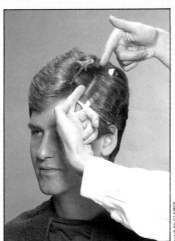

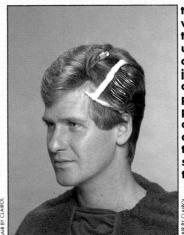

the roots of the hair. This will help protect the hair that is to remain untreated as it will lift it off the section that has just been lightened. The colourist works up to the parting, then repeats the process on the other side of the head, first working on the hairline section, then on the horizontal sections on the side and top of the head

The colour is applied with a wide-toothed tinting comb. It is combed through the first section, which is taken parallel to the front hairline and 5mm into it from the parting. The colour is combed straight through from the root to point. The next sections are taken parallel to the parting, about half way down the head. After the colour is combed on, a small strip of cotton wool is placed at

1 Before. To add more texture and colour to fine, light brown hair, thin highlights will be put through, using the weave/Easi-meche technique

2 Take a fine section of hair, weave out strands and, after peeling back the clear sheet, place the opaque side underneath (as close to the roots as possible). Stick hair to the blue adhesive strip, which will hold it in place

3 Mix Platin Eclair with 30-volume oxidant and apply to hair from just above the dark blue adhesive strip. Place edge of clear sheet slightly above blue line and seal in a downwards movement at edges only

4 After the whole head has been highlighted, leave to develop for 35 minutes (you can see at a glance how the colour is taking because of the clear top sheet). Shampoo, then condition hair

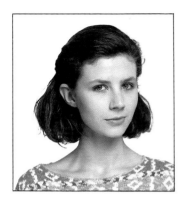
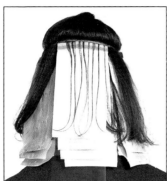
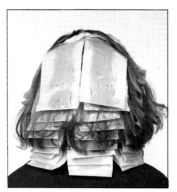
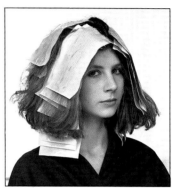

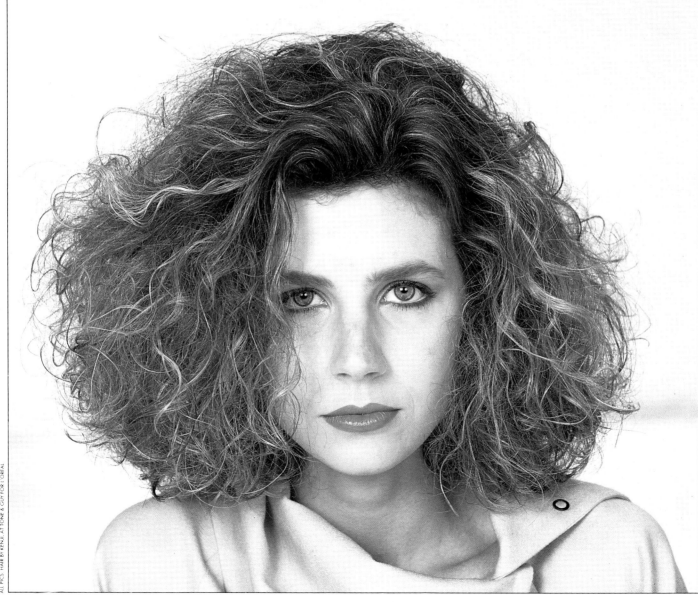

Perming

Today's perms aim not for a rigid waffle-iron effect but for softness, bounce, volume and movement. They are especially useful for fine straight hair that lacks body. If you covet a tight curl you can still have it, but without dryness, frizz and breaking hairs. There is also a new curly perm for black hair that brings softness and regularity to wayward and wiry curls.

Modern perms, used properly, should leave your hair shining and lustrous, but perming is nevertheless a chemical process that alters the structure of the hair and is therefore potentially damaging to it. Because of the necessity for exact timing and correct choice of perming solution — it comes in varying strengths — it is wise to go to a salon instead of attempting to perm your hair at home. If you do perm your own hair, make sure you follow the manufacturer's instructions to the letter.

The perm is a two-stage process. The first lotion applied is a chemical that softens the structure of the hair; this is then rinsed away very thoroughly and the second lotion is applied. This is a neutraliser that sets the hair into the new position determined by the curling rods. A final rinse and the perm is complete.

You should not perm damaged hair. Don't perm and tint within the same two weeks, and don't perm if you have an irritated scalp. Always take great care of permed hair, using a conditioner each time you wash. Avoid brushing if possible, as this will pull out the curl. If you have a wash-and-wear curly style, try to let your hair dry naturally and run your fingers through it as it dries for a soft bouncy look. Use a wide- not a narrow-toothed comb. If your hair looks a bit squashed after you've slept on it, spray it with water from a plant spray and it will spring into shape.

Straightening

This is a very drastic process, and very different from perming. The structure of the hair is altered, but the hairshaft is stretched before being set into its new shape — and this is where the damage is likely to occur because hair breaks very easily if it is stretched when wet. Because black hair is by nature brittle and porous, straightening should be carried out only in a salon. Remember that as new curly hair grows the straightened hair will look less natural — perming is a more successful process as the weight of the hair as it grows softens the curl.

This natural looking perm has given body to fine hair. Scrunch drying with gel creates a carefree tousled look

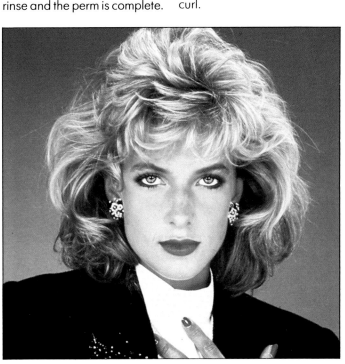

A softly curled perm for a sophisticated look. The perm has given height and fullness to shoulder-length, layer-cut hair. Highlights emphasise the bounce of the curl

The model's long hair has been given a curly perm. It is layer-cut for easy manageability and to give a tapered rather than a pyramid shape. The curls are teased out for a fluffy corkscrew effect

This pyramid cut shows off the abundance of the model's pre-Raphaelite perm, and her hair has been tinted the golden red traditional for the style

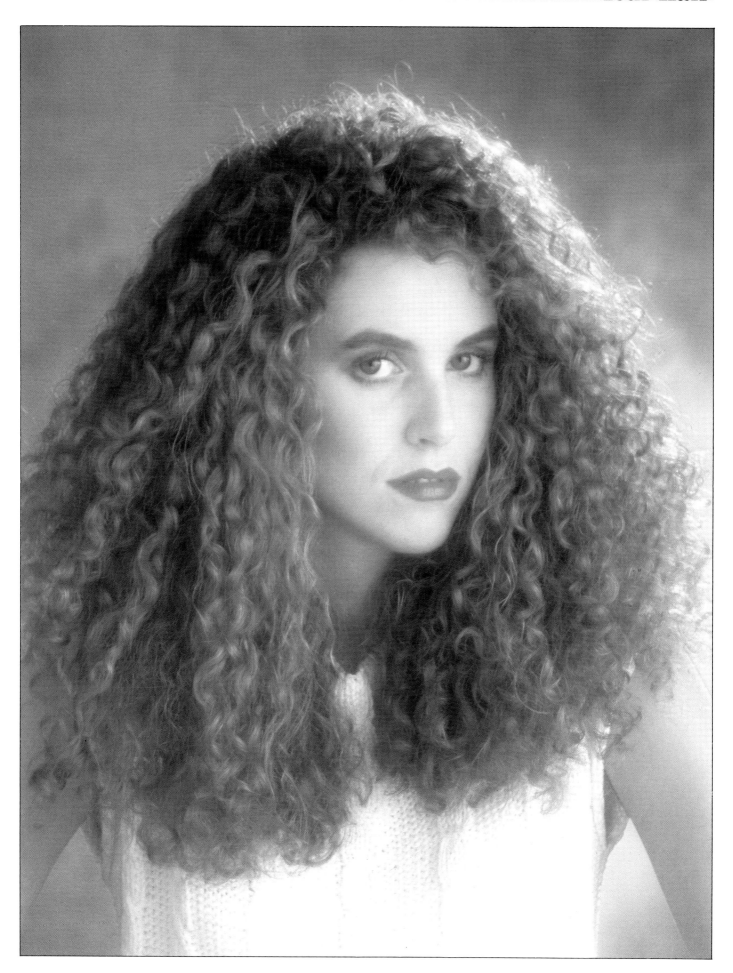

Hair Styles

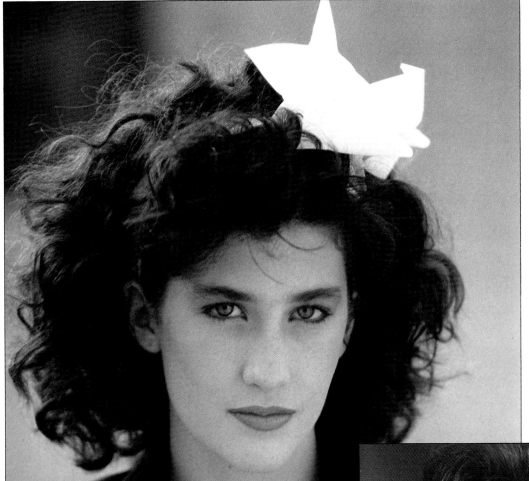

The model's thick medium-length hair was layer cut, lightly permed and then trimmed again to give it a natural exuberance. The curls escape in confusion from their jaunty ribbon for a look that's both sporty and glamorous. An example of how an untamed hairstyle can complement a demurely youthful face

Another untamed look this time combined with the formal elegance of diamante chandelier earrings, a plunge-necked dress and sophisticated make-up, to create a sultry evening look. The model's hair has been softly feathered around the face, but remains full and heavy at the back. The highlights emphasise the movement of the hair. A good dramatic style that needs a minimum of looking after

HAIR BY STEVIE BUCKLE SALON

A longer, fluffier version of the urchin look — a sort of punk Elizabeth Taylor. The feathery cut has been given a lift with a light bouncy perm. Styling mousse combined with scrunch drying results in a carefree windblown style

This haircut was created by triangle sectioning to achieve a very natural look. The colour was painted on, using the tri-light technique, to underline the fall and swing of the style. Use a mousse or gel and a light hairspray to keep this style in shape

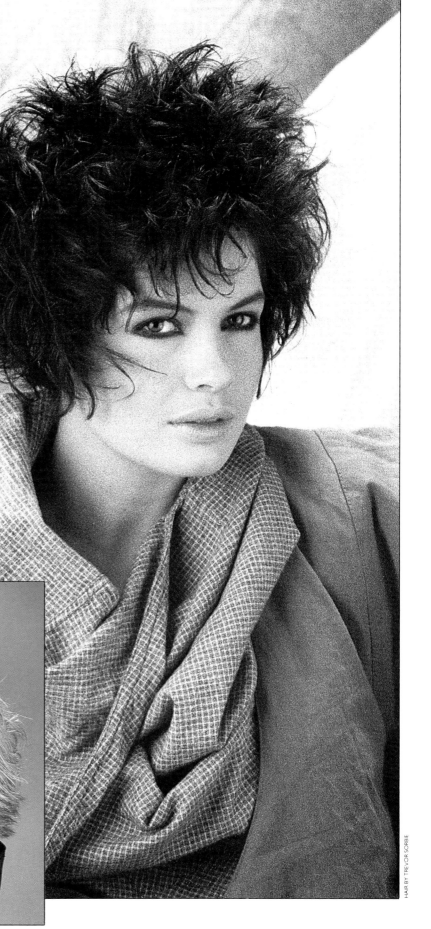

Soft fine hair cut at jaw level is given shine and manageability with mousse. The hair has been finger-dried for maximum textures and highlights accentuate its gentle movement

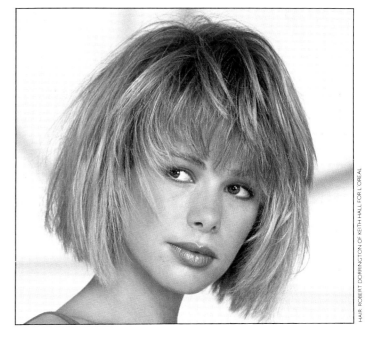

HAIR ROBERT DORRINGTON OF KEITH HALL FOR L'OREAL

Fine hair has been given a light perm and finger-dried with gel for this romantic look that accentuates the model's impish features. An easy-to-care-for style on a soft blonde tint

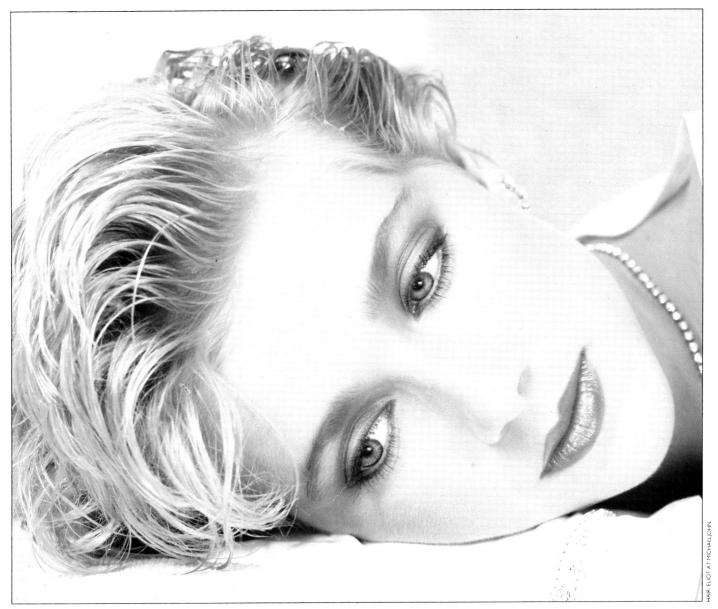

HAIR ELIOT AT MICHAELJOHN

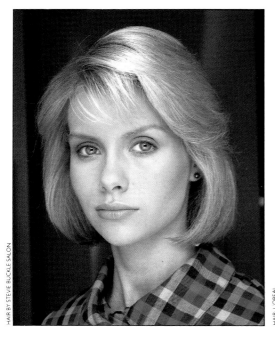

HAIR BY STEVIE BUCKLE SALON

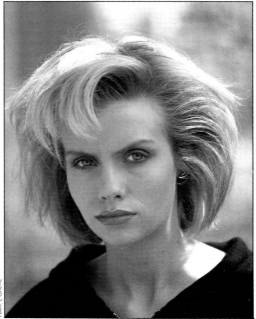

HAIR L'OREAL

Another style on the same hair as top left, but this time smoother and more sophisticated. The model's hair has been deep-conditioned after subtle highlighting. Blow drying completes the natural effect

The same model and a third style, showing the versatility of a superb jaw-level cut. Blow drying combined with hair gel gives her fine hair body and fullness and a carefree sophisticated style that will take her through the day

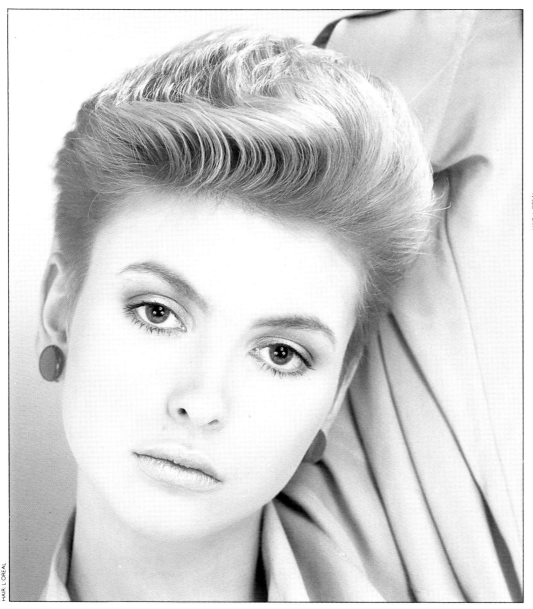

HAIR L'OREAL

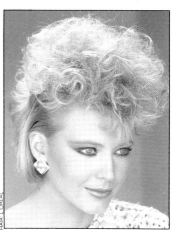

HAIR L'OREAL

A slightly longer style with plenty of froth on top, achieved by scrunch drying on hair gel. The airy curls enhance the golden tint of the hair and the sleeked-down sides give the model's face added height

Short fine hair with a smoother look. Softly upwards-brushed, this style is both simple and elegant. The model's cool make-up reflects her poise

USING STYLING MOUSSE

1 When you have washed and conditioned your hair, squeeze it gently in a towel, then comb or finger through. Fingers are best for permed hair like the model's, but if you use a comb, choose a wide-toothed one. Shake the aerosol can of styling mousse and squirt some into the palm of your hand

2 Taking a little mousse at a time, scrunch it into your hair until you have covered your whole head evenly, from tips to roots

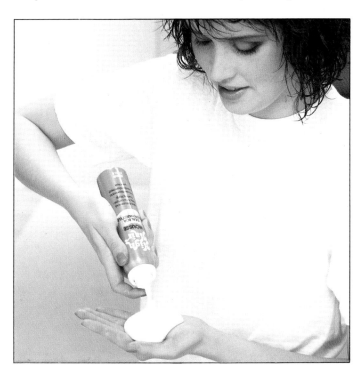
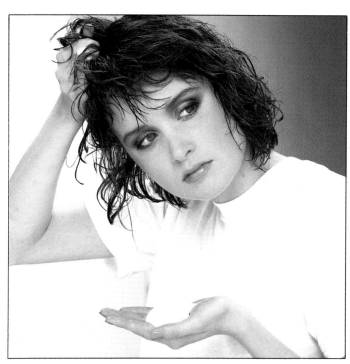

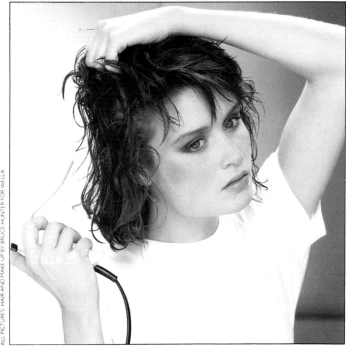
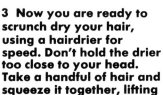
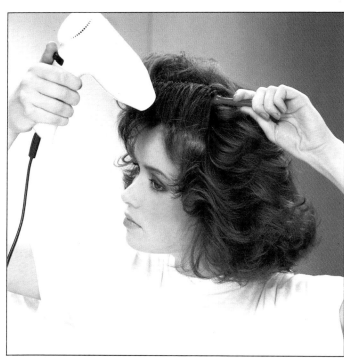

3 Now you are ready to scrunch dry your hair, using a hairdrier for speed. Don't hold the drier too close to your head. Take a handful of hair and squeeze it together, lifting at the roots. Point the drier at it in an upwards angle. Carry on doing this all over your head until your hair is dry

4 The alternative method, which gives you greater control, but looks just as natural, is to blow dry with a brush. Starting at the nape of the neck, roll the hair round the brush and lift at the roots. Aim the drier at the roots and follow along the hair shaft. Continue this process, working round the sides of the head to the top, and finish with the crown

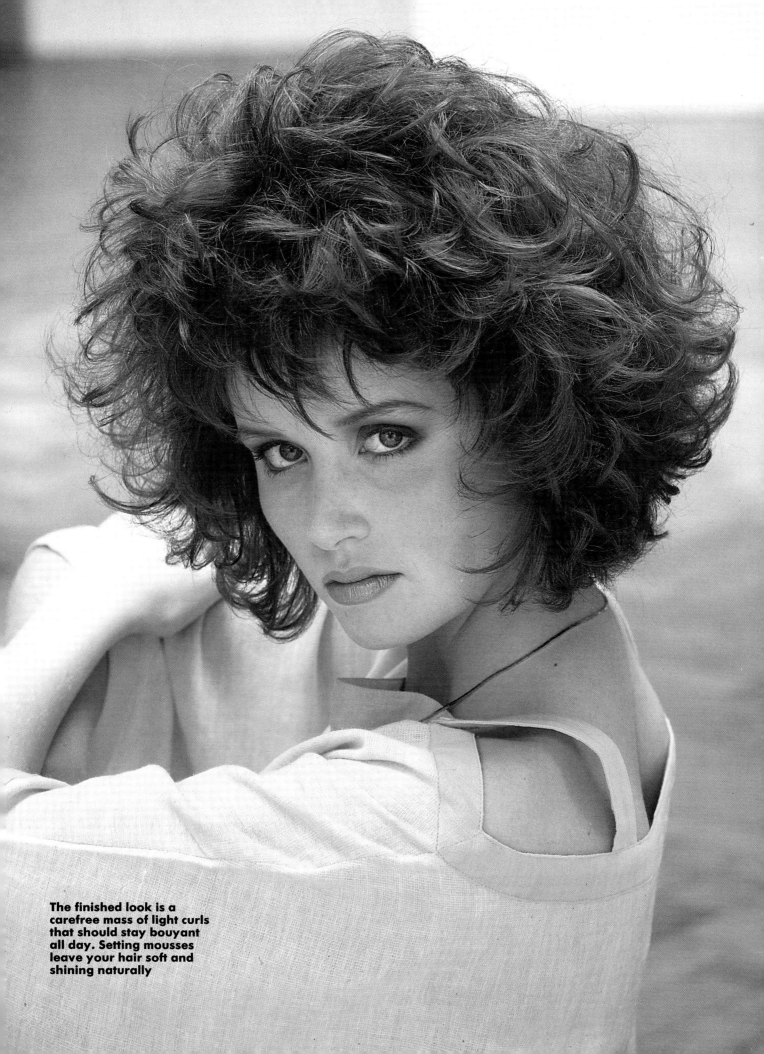

The finished look is a carefree mass of light curls that should stay bouyant all day. Setting mousses leave your hair soft and shining naturally

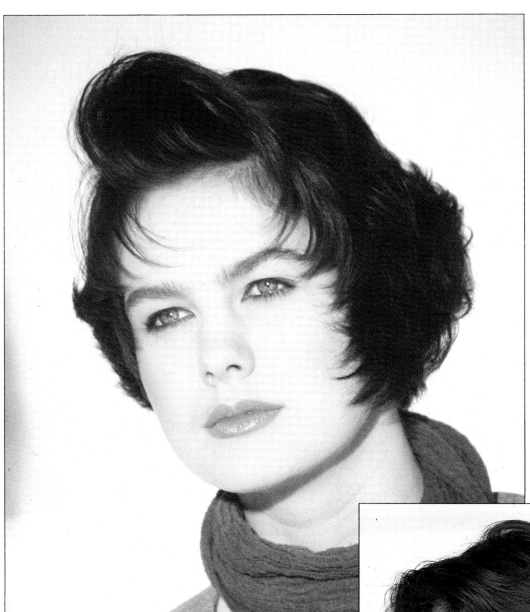

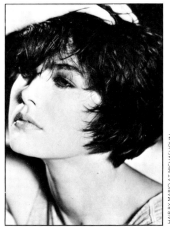

A good cut on hair that's in superb condition. This tousled style needs only a blow dry or a scrunch dry to make it look its best. Ideal for a busy or sporty life, it's a cut that will suit hair of a fine or medium texture (above)

For the best results, this jaw-length style should be blow dried, to create maximum fullness at the back. The soft, flyaway shape complements the model's neat features (below)

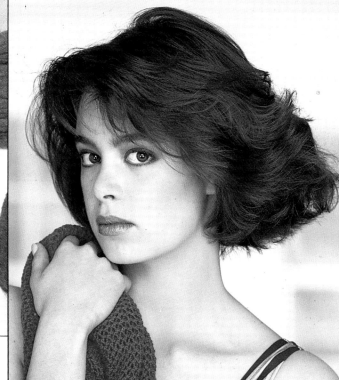

Short fluffy style with bounce on top that fronds forward softly and slims a full face. A gentle styling mousse will help the hair stay as you want it — use curling tongs to create the loop effect on top (above)

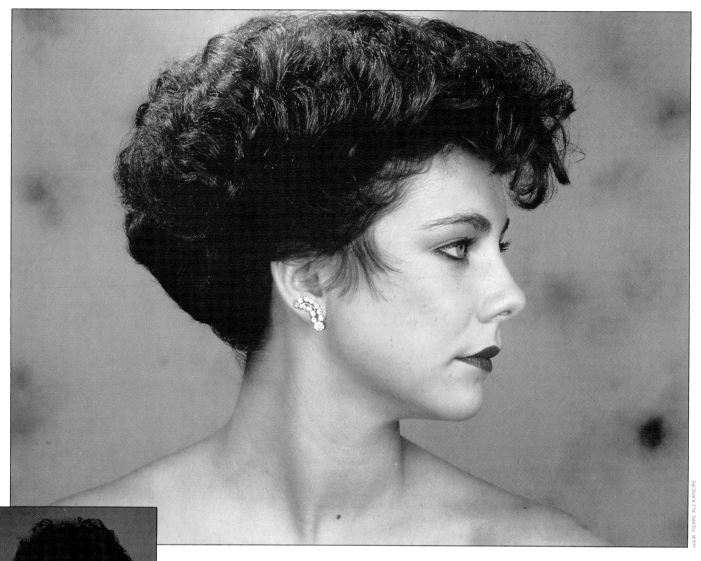

HAIR PIERRE ALEXANDRE

Two ways with the same cut — a curly, casual style for day wear suits the model's outgoing personality. For evening, skilful blow drying transforms her tousled locks into a sleek, sophisticated and artfully sculpted style. An expert cut on thick curly hair gives amazing versatility

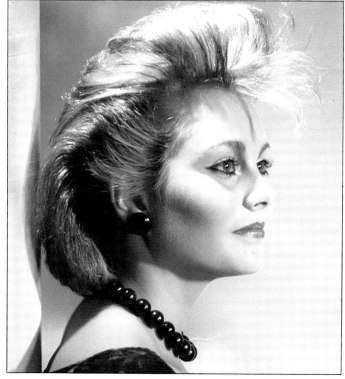

HAIR PIERRE ALEXANDRE

The model's fine straight hair has been wet-set with rollers for evening wear. Brushed up dramatically at the sides, it escapes from its rigid outline in a wispy coif over the forehead. Pink streaks lend an air of frivolity to this original look

This classic bob is a beautiful easy-to-manage style for straight heavy hair that is shining with health. It needs expert and regular trimming to keep its clearly defined geometrical shape. The wearer will always look and feel immaculate

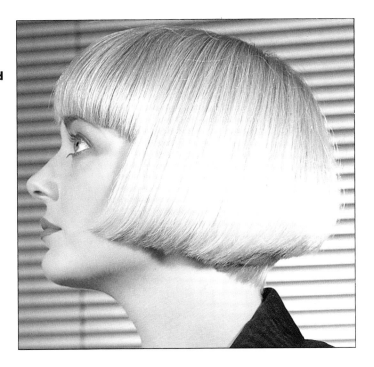

The model's fine soft hair droops limply around her face. She is transformed with an unusual style called the swan line. The hair is lifted up and away from the face at the sides and back in graceful curves, giving otherwise lifeless hair plenty of texture and movement. The style is held in place with gel and a gentle spray and shows off the model's delicate features

A shaggy cut on heavier hair that has been scrunch dried with gel. The hair is allowed to tangle over the forehead, creating a savage jungle look

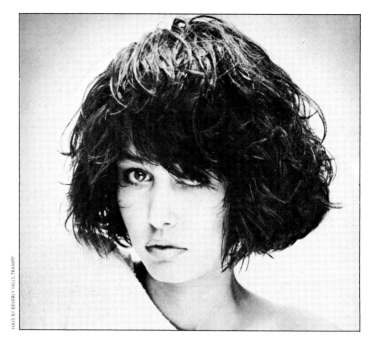

HAIR BY BEVERLY HILLS TRAMPP

A profusion of curls created by scrunch drying on gel — a style to give lift and fullness to fine hair. The hair has been lightened and highlighted to give extra softness

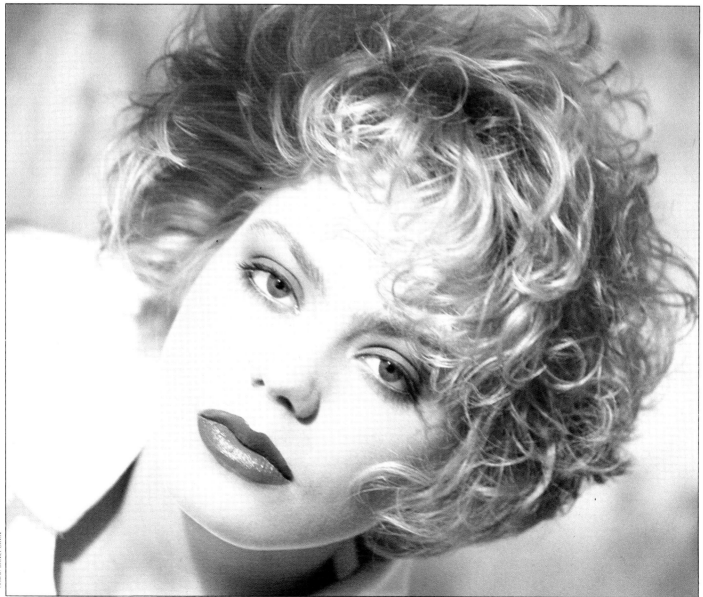

HAIR BY DANIEL GAVIN

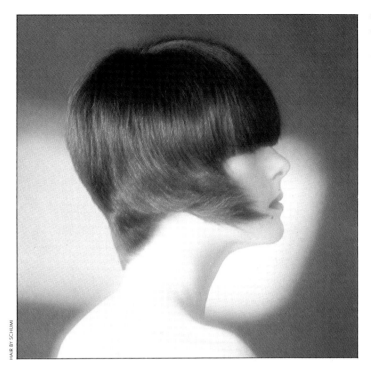

The shingle. The heavy fringe and side hair are given a surprise ending with a feathered edge that fronds forward onto the cheeks. The back is tapered neatly into the nape

HAIR BY SCHUMI

A short cut that needs very little attention — in fact it can be combed into shape and simply left to dry. Layer-cut for fullness on the top, it is cropped over the ears but left longer at the back to curl jauntily round beneath them

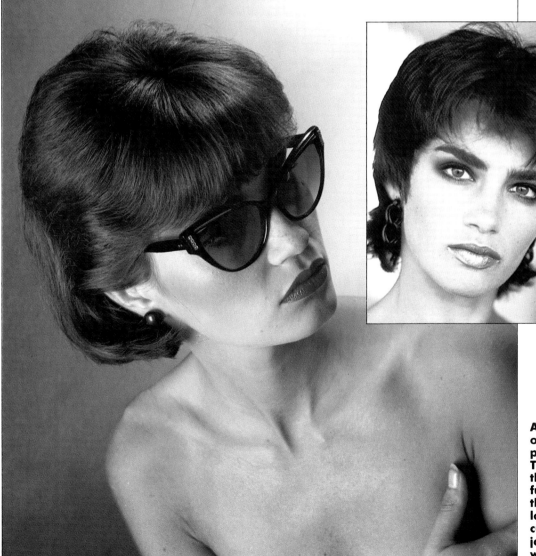

HAIR BY SCHUMI

HAIRCUT VIDAL SASSOON

A neat helmet shape shows off the shine of the model's perfectly conditioned hair. The top hair springs from the centre of the head in a full-fringed bob, but over the ears the hair is left longer and brushed back, curling under at the jawline. A classic cut, dried with mousse

34

An unusual cut with the top hair left long and sleeked back and the hair above the ears cut very short for a raised sideburn effect. Black hair has been streaked with red for a dramatic look

A long shaggy cut that can be finger lifted as it dries. Use gel to create body and fullness. Highlights add texture and interest

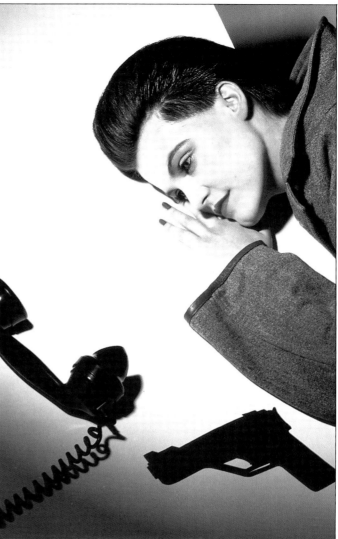

HAIR BY ANDI FOR ANTENNA

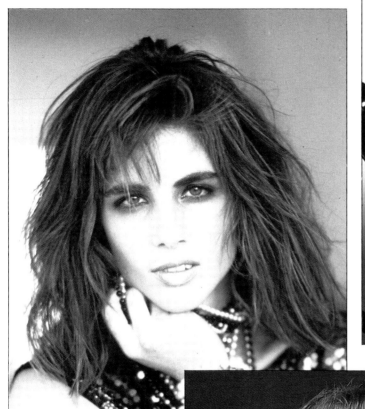

HAIRCUT VIDAL SASSOON

A sophisticated look for evening on shoulder-length hair. The side hair is taken smoothly back and the top hair lifted up and slightly to the side, where it is secured in the centre of the head. A sleek style to show off hair in good condition

HAIR BY SAM McKNIGHT

An easy style for fine hair, cut short at the sides with fullness on top. Highlights add interest. Apply hair gel and scrunch dry the hair to create maximum movement

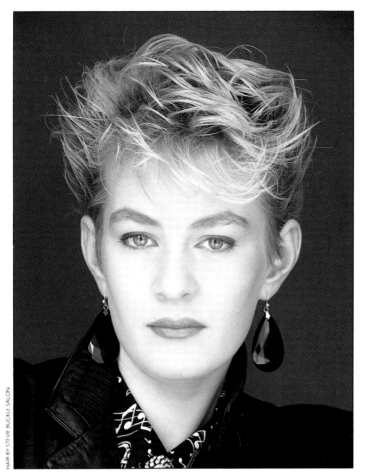

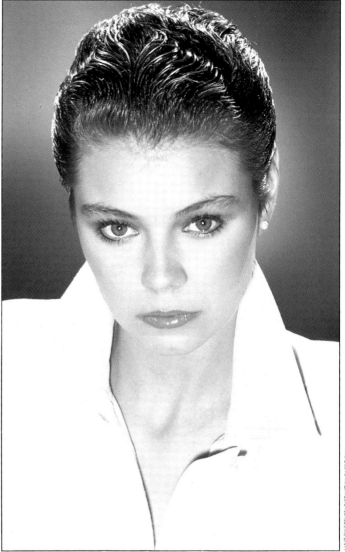

Curly hair can look sleek with the application of a modern hair oil. The hair is cut very short and combed back from the face for a cool svelte style that will take you anywhere — beach, office or nightspot

This avant garde look, reminiscent of Bowie, is achieved with hair gel. The longer hair is slicked back into a ponytail and the shorter front hair brushed up into a bushy coif

The sides have been cut in triangular sections as a more elegant alternative to sideburns. The front hair is left textured and the back cropped close to the head, allowing for a soft and wispy outline, for a look of stunning simplicity. The style is held in place with oil hair mousse

A smooth sophisticated style that gives body to fine hair. The hair is wet-set then brushed up and back over the ears. A wispy fringe can be pulled forward to soften the effect

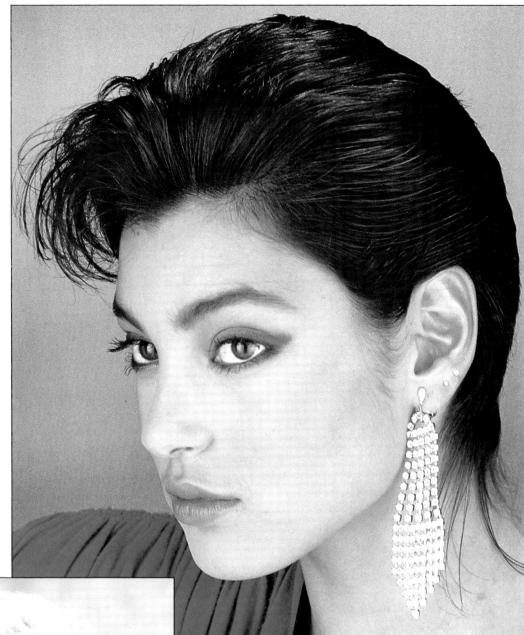

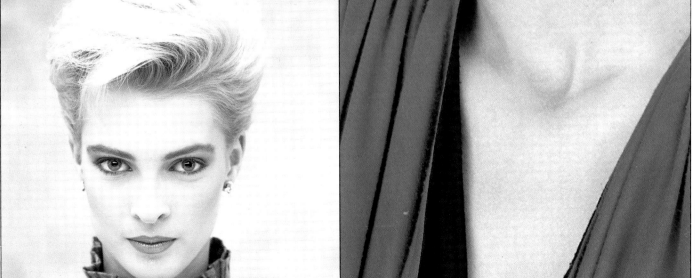

HAIR OSSIE RIZZO AT SANRIZZ

HAIR CLAIROL

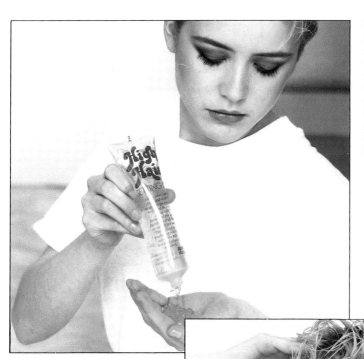

USING HAIR GEL Hair gel allows you to create a more dramatic style than you can achieve with mousse. You can make your hair stand up and do spectacular tricks. It is especially good for creating a spiky, punky look. First, squib some gel into the palm of your hand

The finished look is as prickly as a thistle, but though your hair is literally standing on end, it doesn't feel hard or sticky. Styling gel gives you amazing versatility, particularly if you have fine hair that tends to hang limp and flat (right)

Rub your palms together so the gel covers both hands evenly. Now knead the gel into your hair with a shampooing action, making sure it coats both tips and roots. If you have long hair, you will need to comb the gel right through the hair to make sure it is evenly distributed

To create this style, start with the hair at the sides of the head, combing it up in a wide arc over the ears, and following the line of the comb with the dryer. To create a spiky look on top, finger through the hair in an upward motion, pulling it gently into stiff peaks. Dry from the roots to the tips

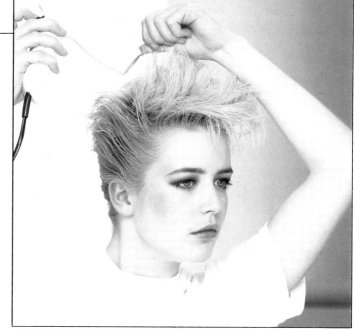

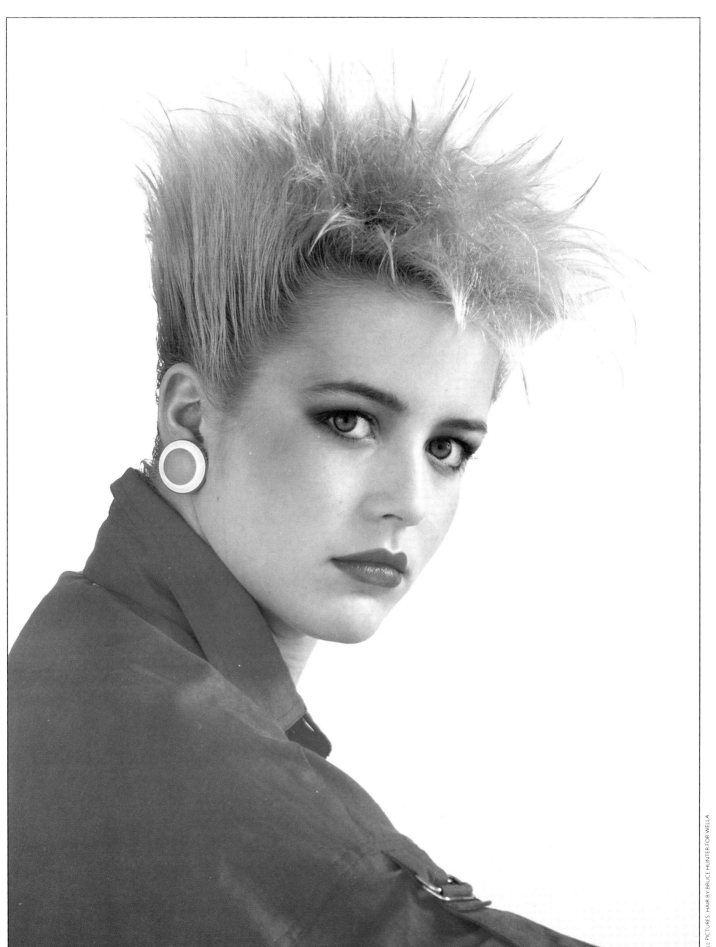

ALL PICTURES: HAIR BY BRUCE HUNTER FOR WELLA

The model's fine hair has been cleverly cut to accentuate the urchin quality of her features. This is a style that's fresh and easy to care for. Highlights draw attention to the soft backwards-sweep of the front hair, while the back is neatly trimmed into the nape

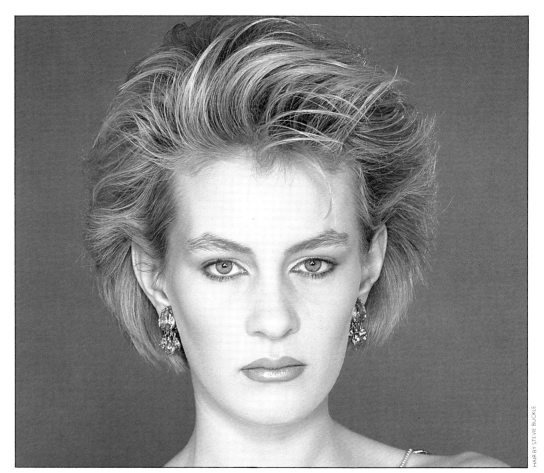

HAIR BY STEVIE BUCKLE

Another soft style for fine hair, this time falling in feathery fronds onto the model's face. The hair has been expertly layer cut from the crown to give bounce and highlights add texture. A perfect, easy-care summer style

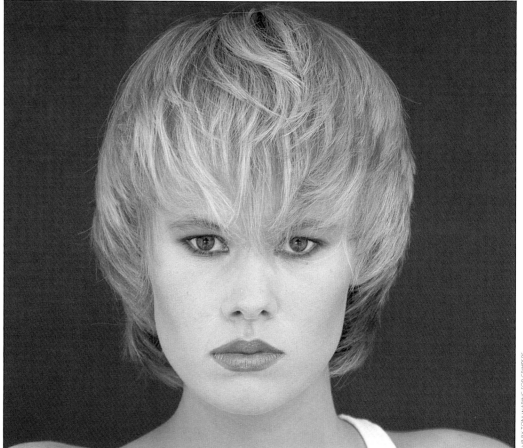

HAIR BY TONI WARING FOR CRIMPERS

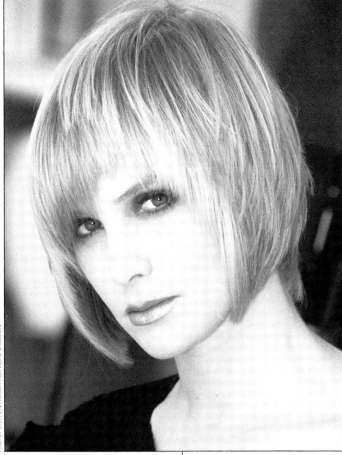

HAIR BY STEPHEN MOODY FOR VIDAL SASSOON

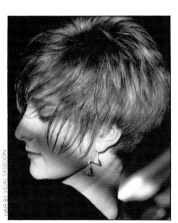

HAIR BY VIDAL SASSOON

A soft bouncy style that makes the most of flyaway hair. Heated rollers have been used to achieve fullness on top and the back has been cropped short and blow dried to stand away from the head. Setting gels and mousses are very useful for giving body to fine hair

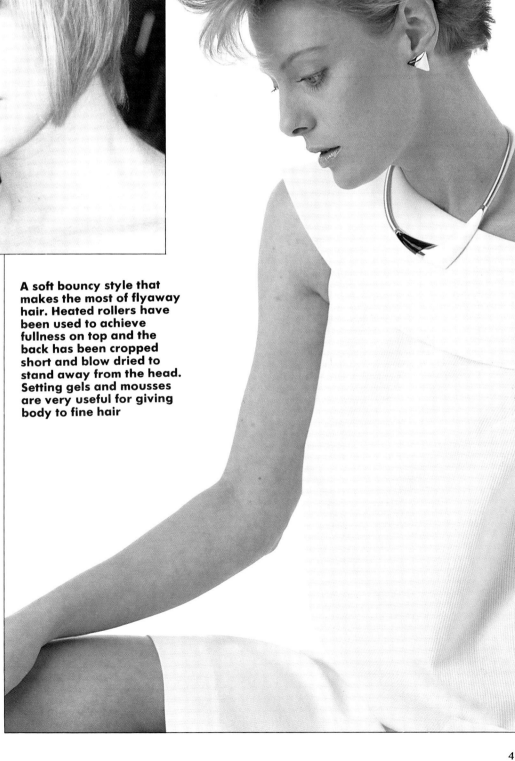

HAIR BY CLAIROL

Fine hair always relies on a good cut. Here baby-soft hair falls forward to create a delicate frame for the face. The gentle curl under the jaw draws the attention away from the heavy jawline to the neatly pointed chin (top)

A windswept layered look whose boyishness is emphasised with highlights. The hair is cleverly cut into the nape to give extra height at the crown, accentuating the model's pert jawline and chin (above)

Long Afro plaits tied with ribbons and beads create an ethnic look for black hair that's suitable for all occasions — and the decoration can be altered to suit your mood. The style takes time to achieve, but once you've plaited it, you can leave it until it next wants washing (below)

A sultry and elegant look that shows off the model's top-condition hair. Height on top and the falling fringe of glossy ringlets complement a delicately shaped face and a neatly pointed chin (right)

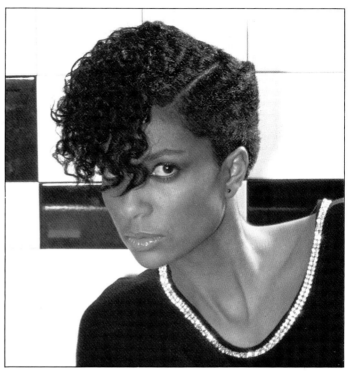

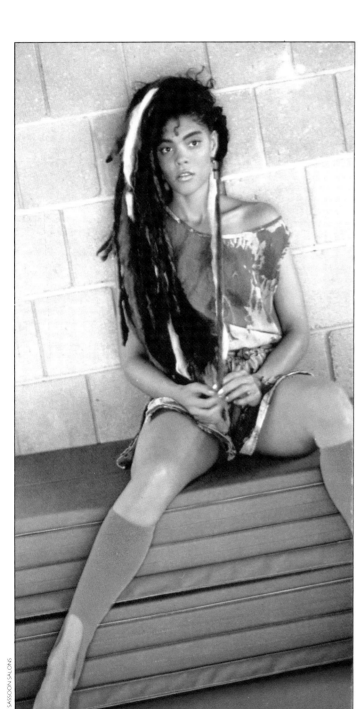

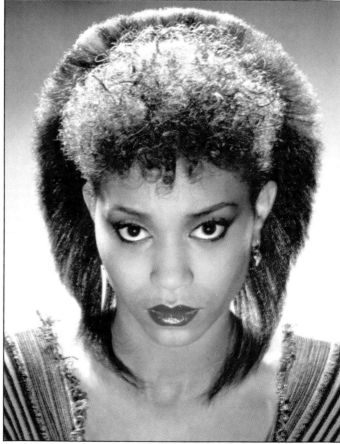

A very dramatic look — almost two hairstyles in one. The top hair has been halo-cut and allowed its natural frizz, while the back has been straightened and cut into a formalised mane. Fun colours have been sprayed onto the hair for a jungle effect (above)

A classic oriental look with a full severe fringe shows off the model's beautiful straight and heavy hair. The geometrical effect is continued with the centre parting and the jaunty behind-the-ears cut to underline the delicacy of the model's bone structure and her long uptilted eyes, dramatised by kohl eyeliner (right)

An oriental look with a difference. A lock of hair fanning out from the crown has been tinted red, for a dressy effect, while a tuft of very short hair at the crown creates the illusion of long hair secured with chopsticks. The hair is cut neatly over the ears and into the nape of the neck (below)

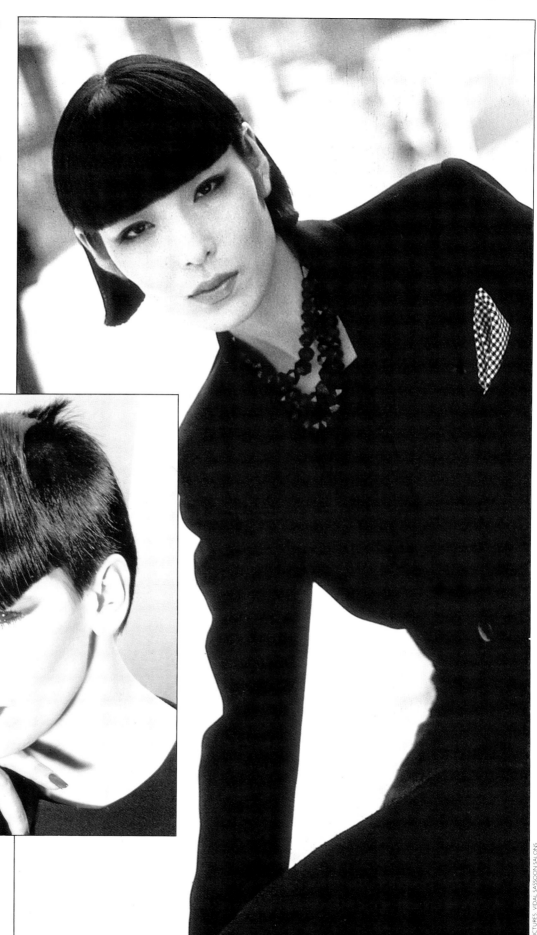

ALL PICTURES: VIDAL SASSOON SALONS

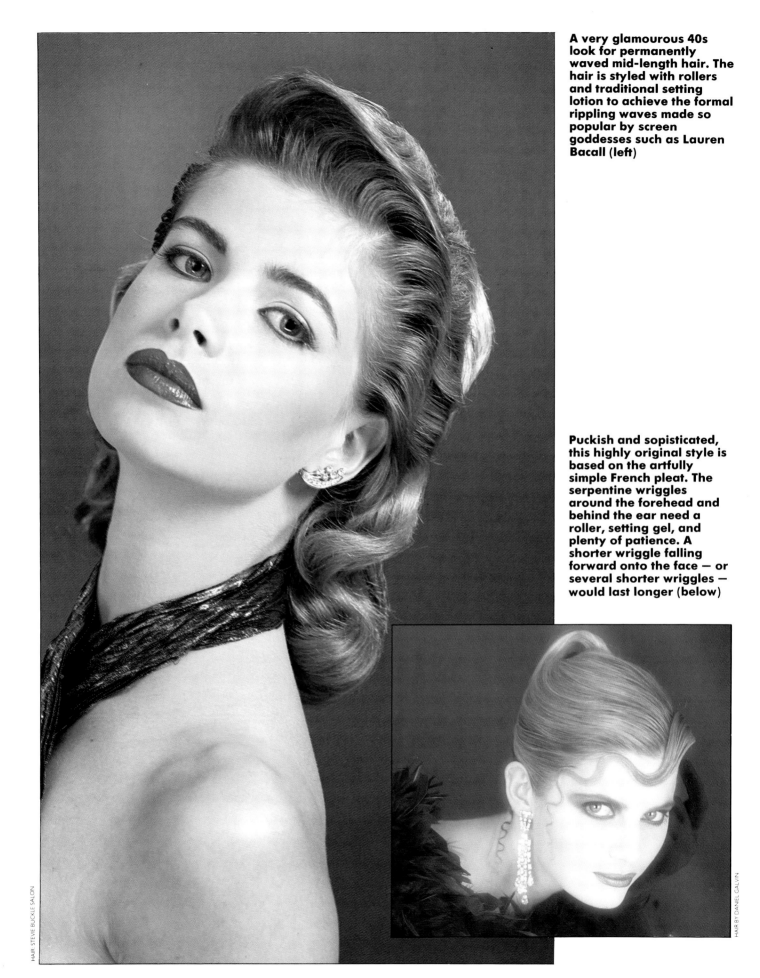

A very glamourous 40s look for permanently waved mid-length hair. The hair is styled with rollers and traditional setting lotion to achieve the formal rippling waves made so popular by screen goddesses such as Lauren Bacall (left)

Puckish and sopisticated, this highly original style is based on the artfully simple French pleat. The serpentine wriggles around the forehead and behind the ear need a roller, setting gel, and plenty of patience. A shorter wriggle falling forward onto the face — or several shorter wriggles — would last longer (below)

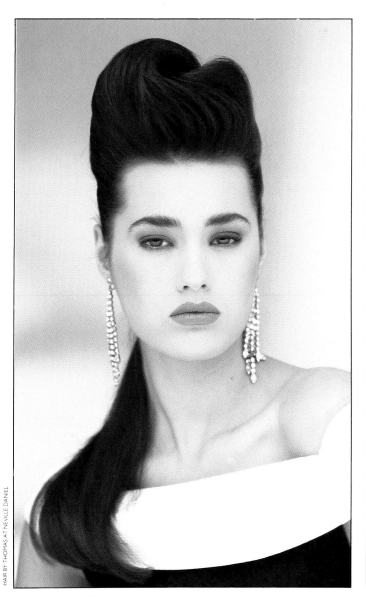

HAIR BY THOMAS AT NEVILLE DANIEL

Oriental elegance. For this style you need plenty of long thick hair. Piled on top of the head in two great waves, and slithering over the shoulder from behind, it creates the impression of cool inscrutability (left)

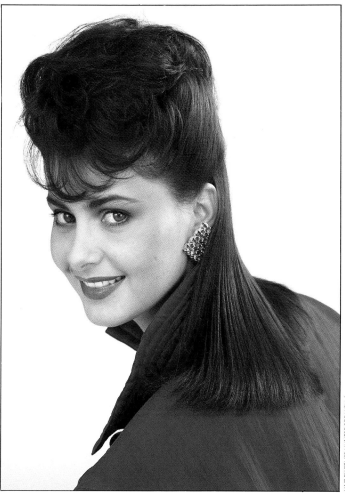

HAIR BY BRUCE HUNTER FOR WELLA

A perfect cut for shoulder-length hair. Set on large rollers and then brushed back and away from the face, this is a look that needs careful attention for formal occasions (right)

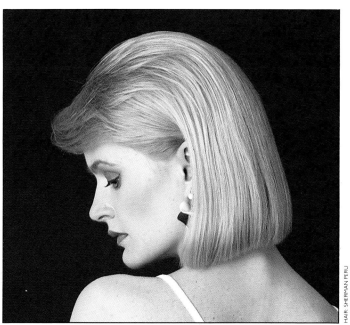

HAIR: SHERMAN PERU

This style harks back to the 50s, when bouffants teamed with ponytails were all the rage. But there is no mistaking today's softer look, with the emphasis on the condition of the hair, and the use of hair gel eliminates the need for too much harmful backbrushing (above)

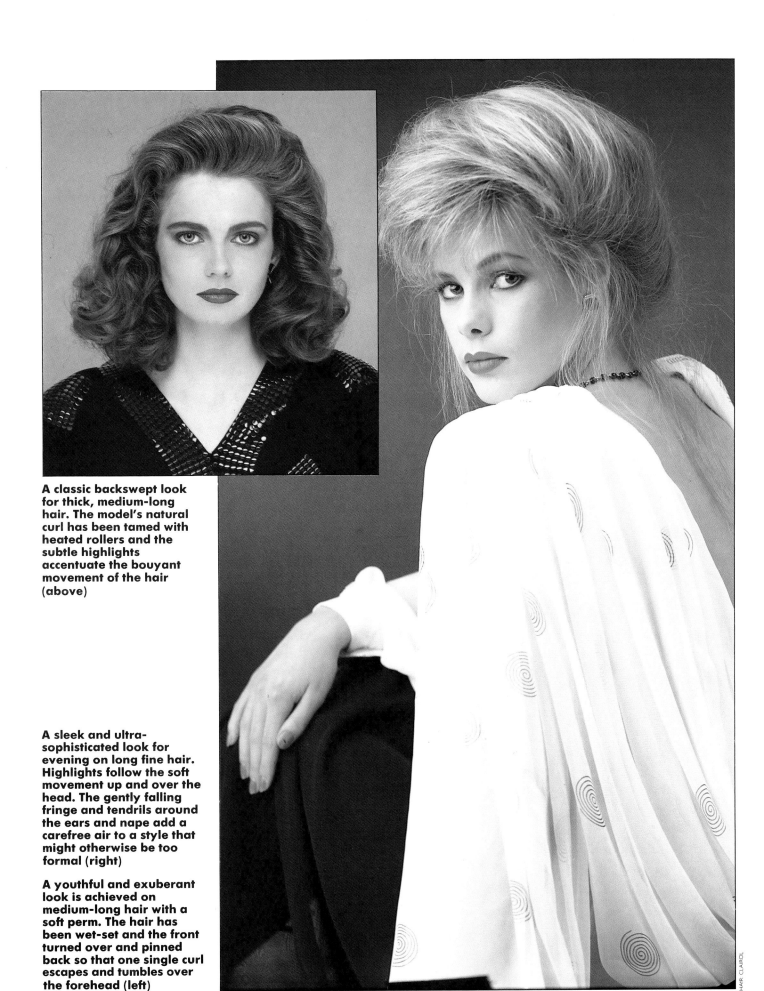

A classic backswept look for thick, medium-long hair. The model's natural curl has been tamed with heated rollers and the subtle highlights accentuate the bouyant movement of the hair (above)

A sleek and ultra-sophisticated look for evening on long fine hair. Highlights follow the soft movement up and over the head. The gently falling fringe and tendrils around the ears and nape add a carefree air to a style that might otherwise be too formal (right)

A youthful and exuberant look is achieved on medium-long hair with a soft perm. The hair has been wet-set and the front turned over and pinned back so that one single curl escapes and tumbles over the forehead (left)

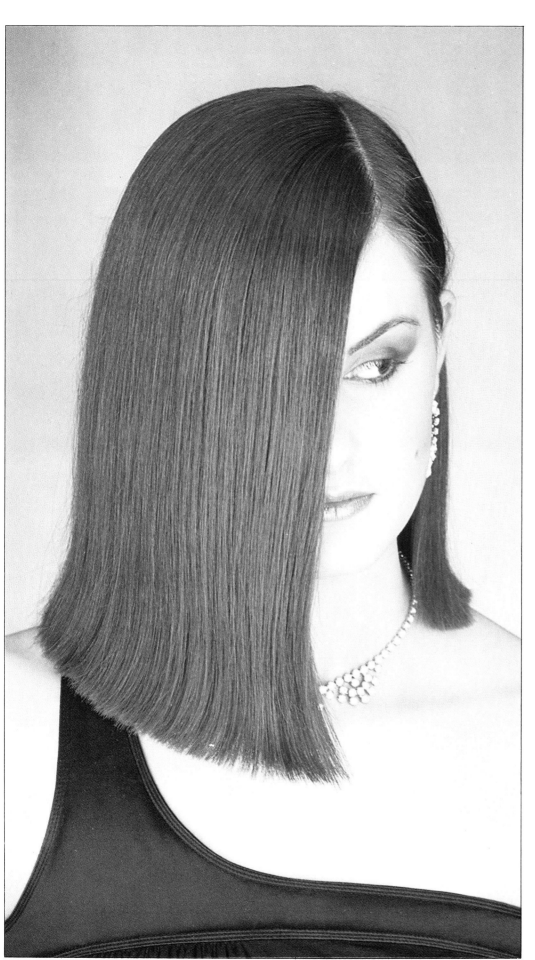

This parallel bob on thick straight hair has fine highlights through the front to give a delicate tone and a look of elegance (left)

Thick, medium-long hair is upswept with a ragged fringe and a complementary ragged topknot — the tails at the nape echo the fringed effect (top right)

This hair has been superbly cut into an asymmetric bob. Its length gives the model flexibility — she can wear it up or down, back, forward, flat or full, as in the photograph. Her make-up is soft and subtle for day wear — for evenings she can add more colour and definition (bottom right)

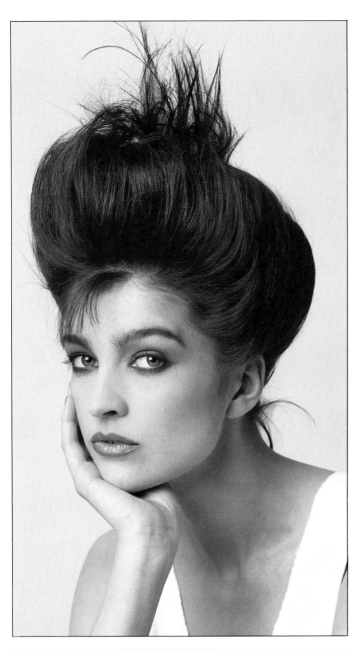

An easy style for thick, medium-length hair. The full, heavy fringe draws attention to the model's almond eyes. The ends of the hair are flicked up slightly in blow drying (below)

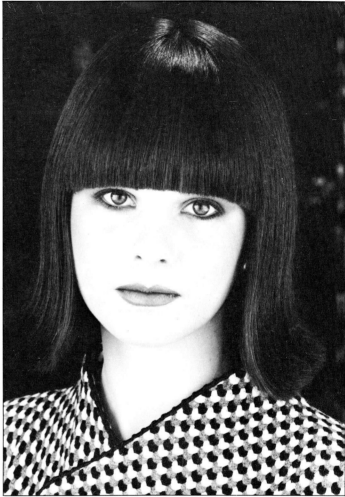

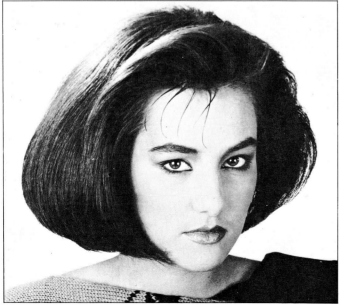

This dramatic look is achieved by roller-setting medium-long hair. The top hair is brushed up and secured in the middle of the head, while the side hair is secured on the crown. The back hair is left to flow free. The style shows off the wonderful conditions of the model's hair

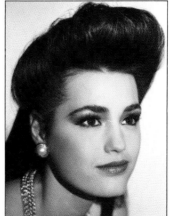